F U T U R E
of HEALTHCARE

Chai CHUAH & Dr H. Omer TONTUS

Foreword by Hon Peter McCardle

For our families

Content

Figures, Tables, Graphics

Preface
by Dr. H. Omer TONTUS

As we know the future will come one day.

Tomorrow, today will be yesterday.

This pre-acceptance applies to all sectors. While changes such as geological changes continue slowly over millions of years, some changes are entering our lives very quickly. Approximately 100 years have passed since the first invention of the phone to portable phones, but it has taken us only 10 years to jump from the mobile phone to today's smartphones. Similarly, in the process of change in health services, while waiting for tens of years for the invention of each new molecule, the period in which dozens of molecules were invented in one year was entered.

In this book, you will find our views as two different individuals who have witnessed the changes in the last 30 years of the health sector. I have worked at all levels of the health system, working both as a physician and a manager in public hospitals, as a hospital owner and manager in private sector, as a faculty member and vice dean in the medical school. Finally, I assigned as general manager in the Ministry of Health and played some role in the policy-makers team. In this way, I have been involved in all the changes and transformations in healthcare for almost 40 years since 1981 when I started my medical education.

The book consists of 3 sections and 17 chapters that are related to each other and cannot be sharply separated. It is easier to talk and write about the past, no matter what. It is easy to do evidence-based and data-based analyzes of the past period, especially if you have a chance to access the written source. However, predictions about the future can be as different as the number of people who can think. It is necessary to use many sources for making predictions. For the better prediction of future healthcare, in all of the book chapters, published articles and analysis of experts were used. As a result, some inferences have been made by using not only our own experience but also the experience of experts in the field of health services.

In general, "The future of healthcare" has two main topics. One is the increasing prevalence of chronic disease and another one is advancements in digital technologies, bioengineering, genetics, the life sciences, and clinical medicine. The first topic is clearly driving gradual increases in morbidity with rising healthcare spending. The second one may lead to improvements in healthcare with the cost. Probably in the short term, insurance companies, reimbursement institutions and governments will face significant spending risk by technological advancement rather than health status changes. These topics are of essentially related. Rising prevalence of chronic diseases is not accidental; it is the results of the investment in biomedical and technological researches.

With these basic approaches, you have been able to follow the changes that have occurred from the publication of the book to the time it reaches your hand. However, we have written our experience based works, which has been going on for years, with the idea that this book will be beneficial for you and for the future of health services. I would like to let you know that we will be grateful for your comments, contributions and suggestions with the e-mail addresses in the imprint section of the book.

I would like to express my gratitude to all contributors, especially editor Mr Chai Chuah.

DR. H. OMER TONTUS
Istanbul-Cardiff
LinkedIn: omertontus
Email: editor@destinationhealthmag.co.uk

Preface
by Chai Chuah

In February 2018, when I elected to finish up as the Director General of Health and Chief Executive of the New Zealand Ministry of Health, it marked the conclusion of thirty-eight years of full-time professional career, twenty-seven of which was in health care.

In those twenty-seven years, I have had the privilege of being involved in many changes in the New Zealand health system. My roles in the earlier years were mostly in financial, logistics, and IT. Ten years later, I held senior positions responsible for managing hospitals and health boards. In the latter years, I made a conscious decision to take up national responsibilities for system strategies and policies. There were many learnings along the way of what works and vice versa. But while in the job, there was never anytime to pause and reflect. There was always plenty to do and even more waiting in the pipeline.

This reality is still valid for many colleagues who are still in the job full time; there is little room to pause and reflect. At a time when all manner of changes are moving at an exponential rate, causing extensive and significant disruption and pressure on the current institutions, both public and private, it is no wonder; health systems globally are facing increasing and growing service and fiscal pressures. More than ever, it is crucial for leaders to pause and reflect, look up, around and far in order not to be lost and consume by the tyranny of the urgent.

Many decision makers today in health care globally, in the face of such pressures, keep doing the same things, sometimes with different labels. These decision makers continue to undertake "reforms and transformation" on a linear trajectory when their operating environment is changing at an exponential rate. Political ideologies, public service machinery of government and private operating models are still pre-21st-century, and would not be out of place from half a century ago.

The growing chasm in social needs caused by the adverse impact of social determinants, pressure of rapid technology advances, and changing communities' demography and expectations acts as pincer movements on many health systems. Yet many health systems continue to tinker with what Einstein calls "doing the same things and expecting a different result."

I have always intended to document my observations and share my learnings. But when I was in the job, this was not possible. Along the way, I kept various notes with the intention of one day, turning these notes into articles. Since February 2018, I have had the time to write a series of articles and posts on my observations of what future healthcare will look like and what it takes to transition towards that future. These are my views to-date and would welcome your feedback, comments, and perspective on "the future of healthcare."

I am grateful to Dr. Omer Tontus for reaching out to me and invite me to join him in this publication.

CHAI CHUAH
Wellington. NEW ZEALAND
LinkedIn: chai chuah
Email: chai.chuah@gmail.com

About the Authors

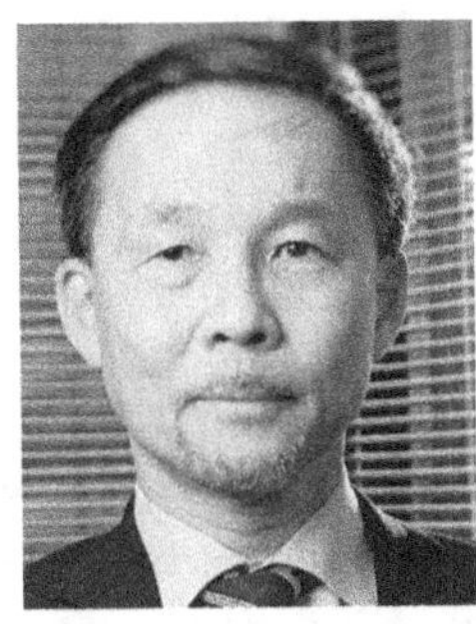

Chai Chuah

Chai Chuah has been a prominent figure in the New Zealand health sector for over 25 years. He is the first Asian to be appointed as the Chief Executive of a major public service department in the New Zealand public service. He has a passion for building a health system together with other partners, which is powered by the needs of the people it serves and which is prepared for rapid changes in technology and demographics. He is focused on driving change in the way the health system works with other public services, communities and other non-public services partners to improve health outcomes, increase access to quality care, improve financial and clinical sustainability, and to develop a unified health system.

After 38 years of full time work, 27 of them in healthcare he took some time to talk, listen, read and observe and think to help him decide his next move. He has been spending lots of time with people that matter to him (especially with his wife), travelling, reading, meeting, connecting and listening to a much broader range of people, writing, started online learning courses and he has even taken up drawing. He is currently focusing on1) contributing and supporting jurisdictions and organisations to transition to a fit-for-purpose future focus healthcare system; 2) help to develop future leaders we need; and 3) research and support implementation of new and better ways of caring for seniors.

He is providing advice to several organisations on the future of healthcare and what it will take to get there. He is also supporting a number of cohorts of talented individuals in their journey to be the leaders we need. He continues to read, think, write and talk on the three areas and would be happy to support any individuals, organisations and jurisdiction on the same journey.

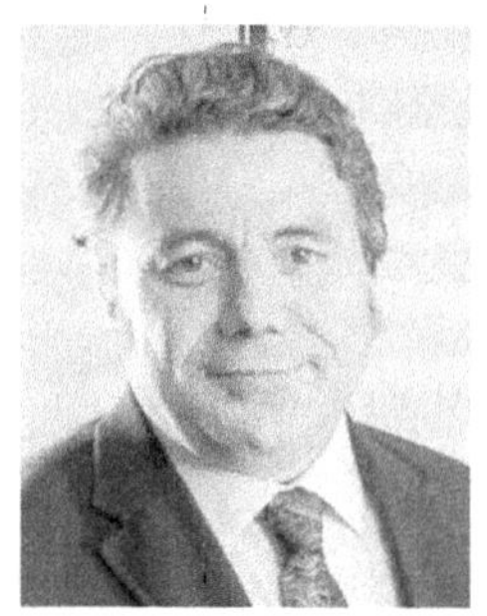

H Omer TONTUS, MD

Surgeon,
Advisory to Rector in Istanbul Technical University
Ass. Professor in Medical Education
Lecturer in Science & Letter Faculty at ITU
Academic Member of Molecular Biology & Genetic Department

Omer is a medical doctor, who specialized in General Surgery and medical education. He attended a program at University of Oxford, UK in general surgery training as an observer. Dr. Tontus has worked in both the state hospital setting and private practices nationally and internationally for many years.

In summer 2011, he started his role as Deputy Dean in Medical Faculty. His main interest was "assessment and evaluation in medical education". He developed an assessment and evaluation software for medical education. Also, he developed a special exam method for clinical period of undergraduate medical education.

In autumn 2013, he started his CEO career at Ministry of Health in the Health Promotion Program for promoting healthy living. He also assigned as CEO of Medical Tourism Department of MoH in 2014.

In Late 2017, he started to work as Advisory to Rector in Istanbul Technical University. In autumn 2018, he started his new academic position in Science & Letter Faculty at Molecular Biology and Genetics Department.
He published 11 books on the topic of Medical Tourism. And he also published many other books such as "Patients Satisfaction", "Event Management", "Principles of Public Healthcare Management". He also proud of his book for high school level students which is "High School Health Information Textbook".

He focused on medical tourism and future medicine, in late 2018. He has been exploring the world of medical tourism and future medicine for a couple of years now and is involved by the interminable possibilities this field is offering.

He also chief editor and owner of Destination Health Magazine which is published quarterly.

His main interest lay in the field of health startups, digitalization strategies for cross-border health and in digital health education. To him, digital health and medical tourism are also key to improve people's health in underserved areas.

Dr. Tontus believes that its time to gather experts' knowledge in all fields and to actively build the future we would like to live in.

He is an antique British silver collector especially from the 17th and 18th centuries. In addition, Dr. Tontus is trying to expand his painting collection which consists of sea and coastal themed paintings of Italian artists of the late 19th century and early 20th century.

Foreword
by Hon Peter McCardle

It is a privilege to provide the Foreword for this insightful publication by two experienced and passionate Health professionals. One a medical doctor, the other an ex-Director General of Health with an Accounting background, whose careers both cover near 40 years in Health at very senior levels.

My interest and perspective is dominantly from a political background; as a former Cabinet Minister in a Center-right Coalition, a leading role in New Zealand's National party 2008, 2011, 2014 and 2017 election Health policies, a member of a Health Board for seven years, and the Senior Political Advisor to the two Health Ministers Tony Ryall and Dr Jonathan Coleman in New Zealand's National Government 2008 to 2017.

These latter years covered the delivery of health services through the GFC. Like all other nations whose incomes had fallen, a deep and sustained examination of options to improve our pressured public health system, under constrained budgets
 took place. Many nations health systems were looked at, not just for best practice in specific health programs but for the health system as a whole.

As a result of this experience, and having been Minister of Employment and Associate Welfare, I am in a position to observe that Health is the most complex and demanding of all the Portfolios. Prime Ministers have observed; if you can handle Health in politics, you can handle anything.

Health is fascinating. How it can be impacted by economic conditions (example Greece and Venezuela), need for constant reforms, balancing stability versus upheaval, and its priorities very much affected by the political change from left to right Governments. In some countries some policy areas are so important there is political consensus, for example, Foreign Affairs or Retirement Income. Such is the range of views on public versus private, socialist versus free-market systems, that few countries have consensus on Health and how best to respond to the simple realities of growing demand due to aging and new health services options.

This publication includes some of the most forward-looking and enhanced Health thinking I have read, and I commend it. It is not a simple read. It very much challenges you to think about the tremendous challenges and changes that are here already,

It adds very much to the future of Health thinking.

Hon Peter McCardle

Section-I:
Future of Healthcare

Chapter I

-

Future Of Healthcare

What Will İt Look Like?

by Chai CHUAH

Health and well-being of people are determined by many factors – genes, culture, living conditions and social determinants. Social determinants influence and are influenced by economic, environmental and political determinants. Health professionals and academics have known this for a long time. There has always been call for politicians, policy makers, funders, providers and health professionals to look at the broader determinants of well-being. After some initial progress especially in public health recent progress however has been ad hoc and slow.

Most First world countries health system now faces unprecedented pressure. In the last few years there is growing concern that this pressure is reaching a tipping point. The convergence of these five main factors could tip these health systems over the edge:

(1) Rapid change in these broader determinants.

(2) Significant societal and demographic changes.

(3) Shift in nature of demand for health services towards more support for life long, lifestyle and chronic conditions.

(4) Continued slow progress to respond to the broader determinants, societal and demographic changes.

(5) Exponential advances in life science, material science, engineering and digital technology.

The impact of the above five factors is fuelling current level of frustration and dissatisfaction of users, carers and providers of current health services as they watch the growing chasm in access, affordability and comprehensiveness of health services.

Reforms and improvements to-date have focus mainly on the "supply" side of the equation such as better horizontal and vertical integration of services, reducing harm and improving quality of services, better and more workforce, facilities and information, structural and organisation changes, more and different ways of funding, incentives, performance measures and accountability.

While some initiatives have focus on appropriate changes in demand, these have tended to initiated from the lens of professionals and providers rather than from the users. The asymmetry of information in favour of the professionals and providers coupled with a more compliant behaviour of the older generation has made some progress in influencing demand behaviours such as smoking cessation. However, there is increasing signs that the impact of the current approach to change demand behaviours is waning. Lessons need to be learnt from non health industries that are more up to-date with influencing consumer behaviours.

Themes of future healthcare

Future healthcare in a 10 to 20 years horizon will have these themes:

(1) Advances in and convergence of digital technology, physical, biological and material science and engineering will drive individualised, personalised and precision medicine. Services in areas of prevention, screening, diagnosis, and treatment are increasingly reliant on insights from rapid advances in gene sequencing and editing. The entire drug therapy research, trials and development process, timeframe and economics will change. The printing of drugs personalised to an individual genomics profile is well within this time frame. Future treatment will focus on intervention at a molecular level rather than the current invasive surgery, radiation and drug therapies.

(2) Big data and advance analytics of traditional health with data from life science, consumer technologies including other non-health data will provide the insights for development of new health services. Initially these new services will focus on wellness, screening, diagnostics and some treatments. Over time such insights will also change most treatment services as we know it today.

(3) Behavioural science (the study of human psychology, sociology and anthropology) will be more prominent in helping to develop future well-being and health services.

(4) New regulatory framework will emerge to respond to privacy, security and efficacy challenges presented by new individualised, personalised and precision well-being, screening, diagnostic and treatment therapies. Technologies like blockchain will likely feature in many systems to respond to protecting privacy and improving security over people personal data.

(5) Players from non-health industries will increase their participation and role in the health care sector. Early movers at this stage are eCommerce tech giants and insurance companies. Other likely new entrants could include energy providers, housing, food, banks and transport. These new entrants are unlikely to enter the health sector by themselves but will do so looking for like-minded partners and reformers from the health sector.

(6) New services, new organisation models, new business models and new partners are inevitable. These in turn will result in changes in the nature of workforce, facilities and technologies.

More & more data points

In the last 12 months more data points is emerging that is signalling the momentum for change is reaching the hockey stick point of the exponential curve. This includes:

(1) The package of changes signalled and underway in NHS England following a very difficult winter has many familiar strands including the call for more funding, more investment I social care, more staff and more facilities. The review of different aspects of their primary care is currently underway including a proposal to accelerate the adoption of a "digital first primary care". The recently appointed Health Secretary Matt Hancock is a Generational Y digital native (he even has his own app!) and his top priorities are workforce, prevention and technology.

(2) Brexit impact on healthcare system in Britain and EU countries is also important to note. One of the main discussion points is poaching and movement of health professionals. Recent articles from England, Ireland and Germany are raising concerns over possible significant post Brexit disruption to their health services.

(3) Announcement of Dr Atul Gawande to head the new Amazon, Berkshire and JP Morgan Chase health venture has highlighted the increased mergers and acquisitions activities in traditional and non traditional health entities such as Walgreens/Rite Aid, Walmart/Humana, CVS /Aetna and Amazon/PillPack

(4) Chinese tech giants (Alibaba and Tencent) and large insurance companies (Prudential, Ping An Insurance) are partnering and injecting significant capital for investment into their health ventures.

(5)   A number of countries funded by National Health Insurance such as Canada and South Africa are under pressure to look at issues of access and comprehensiveness of their coverage.
(6)   The recent data breach of 1.5 million patient records in Singapore highlights the need for cyber security as health system moves rapidly to a digital environment.

(7)   Health and social care system in aged society (Australia, New Zealand, UK, USA, France and Taiwan) are struggling to care for their seniors and is an even bigger challenge in the super aged countries like Germany and Japan. Some forecast that by 2030 (12 years away!) 34 countries will become a super aged society (21% or more above 65 years) including New Zealand.

Transition & collision of the new and old world

Creating a future healthcare system requires an approach that starts by imagining the future and work backwards in terms of what needs to be done. Imagine what future health care will be like in 2030 (12 years away) work backwards and imagine what it will look like in 2025 and 2020. Come up with an agile plan of what needs to be done in 5 years, 1 year, 1 month and 1 week. Mistakes, pauses, u-turns and de-tours are to be expected but each of these provides insights towards progress. A link on an example of a future back approach can be seen on this link -

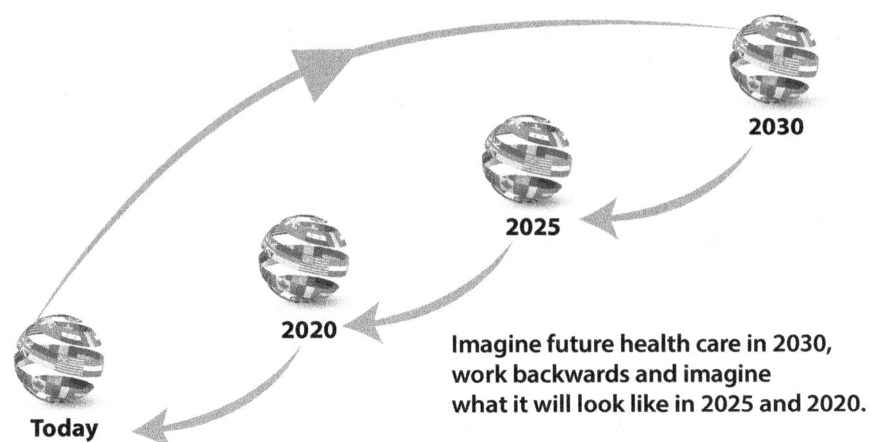

Figure 1 - Imagining the future and work backwards
Adobted From: www.thegeniusworks.com

Current health organisations that will emerge in this future health system would have adopted an implementation that retain and strengthen the relevant core services AND create new services and products. Different thought leaders have written on this theme for example ADAPTIVE SPACE by Michael J. Arena and DUAL TRANSFORM ATION by Scott D. Anthony, Clark G. Gilbert and Mark W. Johnson. Successful implementation of such approach will requires different mind-set and capabilities.

The transition from where most current health systems are today to where they will be in the future will be difficult, challenging and disruptive. The inevitable collision between the slow decision making process and reluctance to embrace change by some incumbents on the one hand and the arrivals of new entrants partnering with reformist health partners is underway.

Two scenarios going forward

There are two broad scenarios of what is going to happen with First world health systems:

In the first scenario some First world health system will cross that tipping point. Despite significant more funding it will experience services failures resulting in negative consequences on people health. This will be the catalyst for change but at expense of people health and well-being.
In the second scenario, decision makers make changes now to create a system that will feature the themes set out above and avoid the chasm. They get to shape the future of healthcare.

The door to be part of the second scenario is open. Accepting this invitation will require an open mind-set, willingness to be part of a team and partnering with new and different type of partners.

This journey starts with accepting that what has been done and most of what currently is being plan (more and different ways of fundng, more staff, more facilities, organisation & structural changes, better integration, better quality and safety) is NOT going to be enough!

There are enough recent literature and publications on how and what needs to be done to transition. These are just tools that need courageous professionals with new mind-sets, talents, capabilities to implement change and a culture of taking responsibility rather than blaming others for these challenges.

Final word

Imagine in 10 to 20 year time what will the population look like, how will people live their lives and when they come into contact with well-being and health services how will they experience it? Imagine what is possible at home, in the community, in primary care and hospitals? One thing is certain it will not look like to-day! So those making decisions today for significant capital investments in fixed physical facilities like rest homes, high street primary care facilities and large hospitals facilities – hope your design are not hard wired and can be easily be re-configured for different uses.

Future healthcare system must address the issues of access, affordability, comprehensiveness and relevance for the users. It must start by imaging what that future looks like and make decision today for a dual transformation to move to that future.

The final word goes to Jeff Bezos, CEO of Amazon reported comments on the Amazon Berkshire JP Morgan Chase ventured headed up by Atul Gawande – *"we said at the outset that the degree of difficulty is high and success is going to require an expert's knowledge, a beginner's mind and a long term orientation"*.

Chapter II

-

Stepping Into The Future?

2 Great Examples İn Healthcare & Education

by Chai CHUAH

I wanted to share two recent great examples of embracing the future. When I read about these two examples, the thought coming into my head was - "some organisations talked about innovation, while others just do it". Sure these are still very early days for both these examples but the organisations working with these technologies are going to learn a lot and will shape the way forward.

Example # 1. Trialling the use of pepper the robot as an "intern" in townsville hospital by queensland health, australia

This initiative will look into the utility of this technology in a ward healthcare setting. The trial is for 5 weeks. This Australian trial now joins a number of other trials in Belgian and Canadian hospitals on how this technology can be part of the healthcare delivery system. This trial should not only be about the technology and its potential impact on the future of work. This trial is an opportunity for Queensland Health and especially Townsville Hospital decision makers through collective learning work on the broader implications for Queensland communities. Dialogue and sharing with Belgian and Canadian colleagues would add to the learning and insights.

Here is the link - *http://www.abc.net.au/news/2018-08-24/townsville-hospital-trials-robot-helper/10157200*

Example#2 . Teaching school children in new zealand school about new renewable energy.

This is a great initiative to demonstrate how a digital avatar interacts with school children about a range of topic on renewable energy (solar and wind power). Watch the interaction between the school children with Will the avatar and watch what happens when the real Will appears in the classroom. The company behind this amazing technology, Soul Machines have numerous avatars for different industries including healthcare.

Here is the link - *https://www.soulmachines.com/news/2018/8/13/meet-will-vectors-new-renewable-energy-educator-in-schools*

In 2038 – twenty year time

Looking out to 2038 (20 year time), such technologies will likely be the norm. No one can stop the future and those who can imagine and embrace the future, gets to shape it. Those that don't, well the future will still arrive and they will still be part of that future but their experience and journey will be more difficult.

There are many questions that need answers and such trials will provide answers to some of them. The challenge is for politicians, policy makers, funders, professionals, providers, unions, employers, academics and civil society to keep an open mind and engage constructively. The reality will be that not all questions can be answered and some will need to be uncovered as these technologies are deployed. The above two examples and other technologies that could have even greater implications like CRISPR/Cas9, the gene-editing technology poses many ethical, moral, security, economic and social questions. In the end, many of these can only be answered through deliberate and careful actions.

How ready is your organisation for the future?

How ready are you and your organisation to make that transition? Have a look at the items on the agenda of your board or executive meeting? Is there any space that looks to creating the future (building bigger facilities is not it!) If all your organisation's energy and focus is on solving today's urgent burning issues, you need to create some deliberate space to discover and imagine what the future could look like. If your immediate reaction to this question is – I do not have time OR I need more resources to able to do the "future thing" your mind-set is already at the wrong starting point. There are plenty of resources out there on the web on this future focus agenda. Here are a few references organisation that have a lot of useful materials that might help (but in the end you have to want to do this with an open mind):

1. Singularity
2. Futurism
3. Forbes
4. Wired
5. McKinsey, PwC. EY, Deloittes
6. HBR and Economist

Clarity of purpose and values driving innovation

Reading and getting an understanding of what's coming is a start but in the end it is the doing that takes us forward. That is why I like the two examples above. The purpose and values of improving well-being, access, affordability with relevance and dignity needs to anchor the call to act. Embracing all the potentially impactful technologies is more than having the first mover advantage or being the first have the next shiny thing. The motivation needs to be driven by using these new technologies to help us solve not exacerbate current global challenges of disparities, inequity, affordable access to education and health care.

The skeptics of innovations often advocate that these new technologies could potentially threaten and widen these societal gaps. The proponents of new technologies need to keep these purpose and values front and center and learn new and better ways to communicate these intentions in their endeavors.

Innovation and its enemies – why people resist new technologies

This book by Calestous Juma is worth reading for those of us interested to understand the issues and the way forward for adopting innovation and understanding why some peo[le resist innovations. There are many excellent points made in the book and two of them in the last chapter is worth noting :

1. "old design patterns are usually not a good predictor of what comes next. Keeping the future open and experimenting in an inclusive and transparent way is more rewarding than imposing the dictum of old patterns".

2. I hope future policymakers will pay greater attention to the disjuncture between rapid technological innovation and slow pace of institutional adjustment.

Final words

There has, is and always will be tension when the future pushes hard against today. Both the incumbent and the innovators have a mutual responsibility not to unnecessarily frustrate progress or recklessly and deliberately put citizens in harm's way. For today's decision makers that are looking up, around and out, and see the future coming at a furious and exponential rate, do not let history record that you were merely observers. Rather you shaped the future anchored and driven by the greater good purpose and values of equity and fairness especially for those who cannot or are unable to speak for themselves.

Chapter III

-

Getting Serious About Making Changes

In Health Care?

by Chai CHUAH

Pressures in First World countries health care system are relentless and increasingly feel insurmountable. Layers of initiatives and services crisscross each other like the picture above. It kind of works but difficult to make change and God bid that it should all collapse one day.

Solutions to-date at best provides temporary relief and at worst actually makes it worst. The mind-set of mainstream decision makers in health care to these intractable challenges is fundamentally to call for more resources (funding, staff, facilities and information), improves the effective and efficient of current services and when it does not work blames someone else.

There are those who realise this hiatus cannot continue and are starting to do something different about this. Some are from the health care sector but it is the non health actors that are taking most of the lead supported by like minded health leaders. While mainstream decision makers in health care continue to discount and put up barriers to these new entrants, it has not slowed down the exponential growth of these new entrants. This week's announcement of the partnership of the UK based Babylon with the China based TenCent together with the current discussion between Wal-Mart and Humana in the USA are the latest data points providing a clear signal of the trajectory of change in health care. These new entrants will not always get everything right and are likely to make some mistakes along the way. But they are more agile, open minded, understand the power of exponential technology, faster to give up what does not work, figure out and try what might work.

Attempts by mainstream decision makers in the health care to-date have not provided durable answers yet more of same is still being proposed in most First World countries. They have not and will not work because:

• Linear and complicated solutions are proposed to solve complex problems.

• Solutions are often design to improve each of the fundamentals e.g. workforce, funding, facilities but not the relationship between them. Such silo approach is actually making the situation worst not better by reinforcing the importance of each fundamental but not the whole system.

• Solutions offered to date on improvements are design to make the current system more effective, efficient and productive when changes in context and environment requires disruptive not sustaining innovations.

• Talents, capabilities and structures needed for disruptive change is fundamentally different from those that are managing the existing system.

Complex rather than complicated or linear

Linear and complicated solutions do not and will not work because complex challenges and problems have these characteristics:

1. There are many and increasing number of causes
2. The relationship between these causes and their effects are not well understood, difficult to explain and constantly changing
3. The cause-effect relationship can only be seen after they have occurred and are difficult to predict
4. Even when the cause-effect relationship becomes apparent after it happens they do not necessarily repeat themselves
5. Data at best provides insights into correlation but does not explain causal relationship (why it occurs)

A **discovery approach** with a portfolio of safe to fail initiatives is the right response to find solutions for complex challenges. Some of these initiatives will not work but learnings from it provide insights for initiatives that follow. If there are no failures then these portfolio of initiatives will not contribute to discover the way forward. There are no best or good practices to solve complex challenges. Yet how many times have we heard comments like "let's not reinvent the wheel and adopt these best or good practices". The value of the discovery approach is more in the learning and process rather than the milestone or results.

Optimising relationships between fundamentals

How many "advisory groups" for workforce, eHealth, capital planning, funding have come and gone and the challenges not just remain but gets more pressing. That is because each of these is design to make recommendations to optimise each of these respective areas. Even when a whole system advisory group is set up, recommendations on these fundamentals are almost always cherry pick by decision makers when it comes to implementation. Current interventions are design to respond to "events" or "trends that emerge from a series of these events" but not the underlying weakness of the relationship between the fundamentals of the whole system.

Complex social challenges need a system approach that optimises the relationships between all the fundamental parts rather than optimise each fundamental part.

Disruptive not sustaining innovations needed

Making improvements (effectiveness, efficiency and productivity) on somethings that works but was design for a different time, context and environment is flawed. These sustaining innovation improvements still have to be pursued. But on its own it is not nearly enough and does not and will not improve access, affordability and equity of health outcomes that has emerged as a result changes in context and environment.

The theory of disruptive innovation introduces new partners, new technologies, new networks, new operating and business models that is more relevant for today's context and environment. These disruptive innovations properly executed will improve access, lower cost that can contribute to improving equity of health outcomes for those who currently are missing out.

Different talents, capabilities and operating models

Asking current leaders whose talents and capabilities are design to manage current system to disrupt themselves is like asking the turkey to vote for Christmas. Incumbent leaders need to keep doing sustaining innovations to create the head room for disruptive innovations. But they are not the ones (no fault of their own) that can deliver on the disruptive innovation agendas.
Likewise current organisation structure, incentives, rules and criteria of success, capabilities, skills and knowledge are all orientated towards managing status quo.

Disruptive innovations require different talent, capabilities and operating models to execute a discovery approach on a portfolio of safe to fail initiatives that strengthens the relationships between all the fundamentals of the whole system. Therefore a dual transformation approach that clearly separates the talents, capabilities and processes of sustaining from disruptive is needed. Can this be done within a single organisation? There is some emerging literature that suggests it is possible but current exemplars from what works in other sectors points to a need to be set up separate organisation lead by leaders with different set of talent and capabilities.

Linking the four concepts

These four concepts are interconnected. Complexity framework recognizes that a discovery approach is the right response. The discovery approach is disruptive and requires a portfolio of safe to fail initiatives that strengthen the relationships between the multiple and varied fundamentals that make up the health eco-system. Different talent, capabilities and structures are needed to take a discovery approach to execute disruptive innovations.

Concluding remarks

As someone who could be serious about making changes to health care take some time to mull over this article and begin the journey to find out whether you are a sustaining or disruptive leader because you cannot be both.
To help you with your discovery journey listen to these talks that explains the above concepts and more (like big data, etc) in greater details.

Video 1 - https://www.youtube.com/watch?v=5h17eUJ-val&t=291s
Video 2 - https://www.youtube.com/watch?v=oHnwq2F6204
Video 3 - https://www.youtube.com/watch?v=p6vkDm50Bh8.
Video 4 - https://www.youtube.com/watch?v=N7oz366X0-8

Video 1

Video 2

Video 3

Video 4

Chapter IV

-

What Is Missing

From Previous & Current
Healthcare Reforms?

by Chai CHUAH

Health organisations are large complex entities

Many health organisations are complex and substantial organisations with significant budgets, employing large number of highly qualified staff, operating and owning substantial facilities and assets. Leading these organisations at the best of times has always been challenging. Increasing and mounting pressure are triggering another round of major "reforms, reviews, transformation" in a number of First world countries (UK, Canada, South Africa and New Zealand)

Reforms to-date have not addressed the pressures faced by First world countries health system. They are and will be temporary band aid because:

- they focused on individual elements like funding, structure, workforce, facilities, integration, technology, etc rather than taking a whole of system approach.
- lack of a robust dual transformation agenda
- there is little or no focus on "leaders we need".

Any reform agenda should have three foundation pillars. First the scope should not only cover comprehensively the whole of system but take a systems thinking approach (as suggested by David Stroh in his book System Thinking for Social Change) . Secondly it needs to have a dual transformation agenda (as set out in the book Dual Transformationby Scott D. Anthony, Clark G. Gilbert, Mark W. Johnson) that re-positioning of traditional core business and concurrently creating a separate new future. Thirdly, it needs look at the "leaders we need" for implementation. There is no point having a system thinking and comprehensive reform agenda and a dual transformation focus if we do not have leaders needed for implementation.

Lesson from a case study in health system reform

One of the great experiences in my career was to be part of a Ministerial Review Group (MRG) tasked with making recommendations (within existing legislative framework) to improve the sustainability of the whole health system. Most of the recommendations were accepted by the government of the day. However during implementation some initiatives made progress while others got bogged down.

Recommendations that struggled with implementation were largely due to the fact that "we did not have the leaders we need to do the job". MRG made a fundamental assumption that the system had the "leaders we need" for implementation. So as I look at several First world countries going through another round of major "reviews, transformation and reforms" I cannot help but feel that the same flawed assumption is being made.

Styles of leadership

Today's leadership model as described by author Michael McCoby is largely "master craftsman and industrial style leaders". In today's knowledge economy characterized by rapid and constant changing environment fueled by a digital revolution these models of leadership are no longer appropriate. Today's challenges and opportunities are far too complex for traditional master craftsman and industrial style leaders to cope with. Their response to today's environment is too linear, slow, top-down and autocratic. What is needed is a knowledge based network leadership model. This model focuses on having a network of leaders capable of working as a team to provide the width, depth, agility and speed in their responses. This model de-emphasizes big personality, and big ego mentality type of leadership.

Complex and complicated challenges

Complex and complicated challenges require very different responses. Often these two words are used interchangeably. The Cynefin framework clearly highlights a seismic difference between the two. Complicated challenges for example can be solved by good solutions developed with the help of experts and data analytics. However, for complex challenges searching for best or good practices or solution is the wrong response. The response for complex challenges is a discovery mind-set implementing a portfolio of safe to fail initiatives.

Therefore these two very different responses need two very different types of leaders with different talent, temperament, skill, knowledge, capability and capacity.

Talent, temperament, skill, knowledge, capability and capacity

Comprehensive reform agenda with a dual transformation focus needs to carefully also look at the different talent, temperament, skill, knowledge, capability and capacity needed for implementation. Often these terms are used interchangeably and there is either confusion or lack of clarity of what they mean. For the purpose of this article let's put some definition around what they mean.

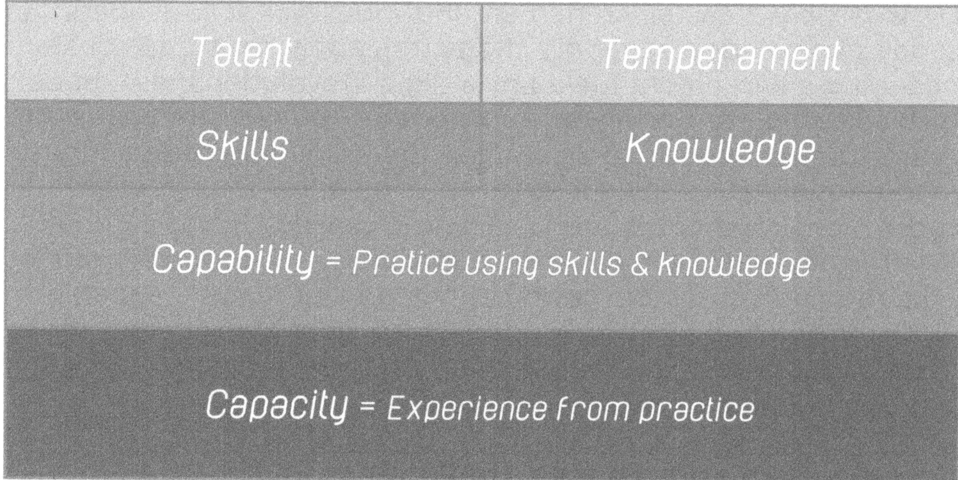

Table 1 - Comprehensive reform needed for implementation.

Talent is a natural ability that we were born with and stays with us. ***Temperament*** refers to our in-born behaviors and emotions we tend to exhibit that remain stable throughout our lifetime. ***Skills*** are the proficiency developed through training and practice. ***Knowledge*** is the theoretical understanding of a topic or subject. Knowledge can be acquired and learned through multiple channels including discussions, workshops, conferences, seminars and academic qualifications. ***Capability*** refers to the ***skills and knowledge*** required for a particular task for example "change management". ***Capacity*** refers to our ability to absorb change or undertake multiple concurrent complex interrelated projects effectively.

For example the team leader and team members leading complex initiatives with high level of fluidity, ambiguity and tight timeframes should have:

1. talent for thinking outside the box,self- directing and decisive

2. calm and positive temperament,

3. knowledge of system and agile thinking,

4. skillful in navigating changing priorities and

5. capacity to drop, change and add new areas of work on short notice

Suggestion for your reform agenda – leaders you need!

1. Make sure there are two distinct teams: one to focus on re-positioning current system and the second to focus on creating the new future. A common mistake is assuming that the same team can do both.

2. The leaders and team members of these two distinctly separate teams need to have the right talent, temperament, skill, knowledge, capability and capacity for the task at hand.

3. Within each team ensure that there is alignment of talent, temperament, skill, knowledge, capability and capacity is also a recipe for disaster. For example, there is no point having a team with the right talent and temperament but with insufficient and inappropriate skill, knowledge and capacity.

Final word

Not too long ago I listened to a talk on "the leaders we need". The speaker outlined an asymmetry gap between the leaders we need and the leaders we have and want. I took four points from his talk:

1. Leaders need to be able to check their egos in the interest of greater good
2. Leaders need to have a shared purpose of greater good beyond their own agenda
3. Leaders need to value team more than any individual especially themselves
4. Leaders need to have courage to take responsibility, learn and act

Any reform agenda where their leaders do not meet the above 4 characteristics no matter how talented, skillful, knowledgeable and capable will not be successful.

Chapter V

-

Addressing Health System Deficits

Changing Structures A Distraction

by Chai CHUAH

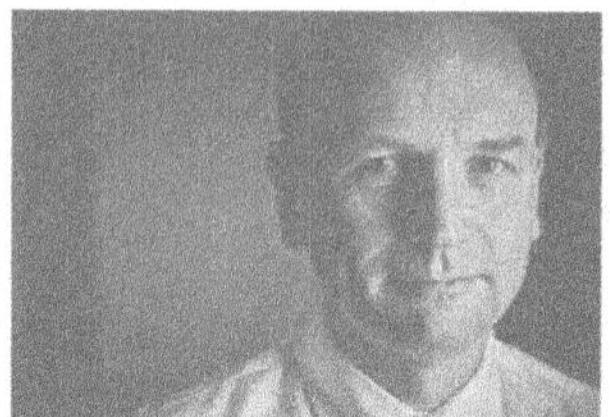

NHS England announces fewer CCGs as part of long-term plan

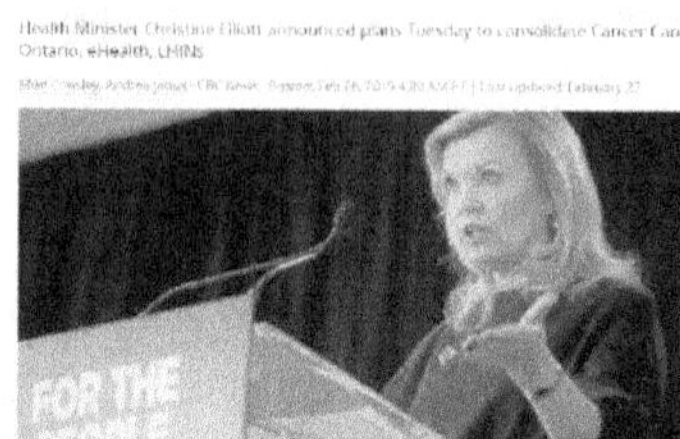

Ford government creating Ontario Health super-agency

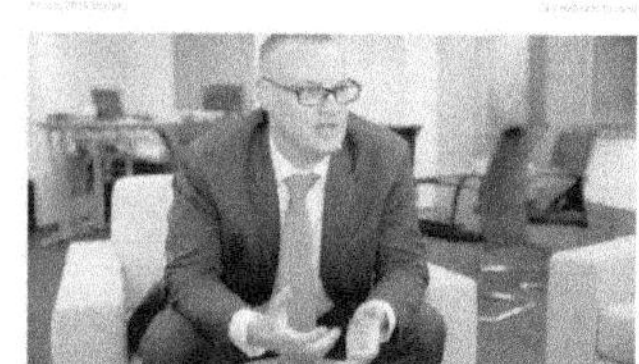

DHB bosses and board members cost taxpayers $65 million a year

Context

First world countries health systems are complex, with a large budget, and in many instances are also large employers. One of the challenges has always been to design system and organization structures to deliver health services. However, when health systems face growing pressure on health services and spiraling deficits politicians, policymakers, health professionals, unions, health managers, and other commentators tend to point the fingers at a mixed bag of favorites which includes lack of funding, and bureaucratic structures.

Many health systems will have a mix of centralized and decentralized organizational structures. When health systems are not performing and come under pressure, centralized structures will be blamed for being too bureaucratic, out of touch, and too slow to respond, while decentralized structures, on the other hand, will be accused of being fragmented, uncoordinated, postcode access to health services, losing the synergy of size, and duplication of resources.

When health systems are not performing, more often than not, there will be other systematic issues which many "transformational" reforms program will attempt to address. However, they are commonly done without addressing the complex inter-dependencies between them. More funding, more workforce, facilities, IT systems, different commissioning models, more integrated delivery models, different accountability arrangements, various performance measures, different governance models are the common elements of a multi-facet reform program. No structures are ever perfect, and when there are performance issues, it may not be just a structure issue.

Here are some realities of structural changes:

1. It always takes longer than plan and creates uncertainty
2. It will cost more money than it saves.
3. It will divert attention away from frontline health services.
4. Many of existing health managers will be re-appointed.
5. It rarely results in changes in models of care at the frontline
6. Risk of worsening performance of existing services is high.
7. Significant proposals waiting for approval are likely to be stalled.
8. It will fail to address sustainability, equity, and affordability issues.
9. It will fail to improve better outcomes and experience for users of health services.
10. It cannot address culture, values, or behaviors and change closed mindsets.

Yet, structural changes are very much part of current health systems reforms. Here are three examples:

1. The new Ontario government in early 2019 announced that they were creating a superagency, consolidating 14 Local Health Integrated Networks (LHIN) and 6 standalone agencies (example, Cancer Care and eHealth) into one super-agency, Ontario Health.

2. In NHS England, an April 2019 GP Online article reports of speculation that the current 190 Clinical Commissioning Groups (CCGs), under the NHS Long term plan will reduce to 44 with 1 CCG for each of the existing Sustainability and Transform Partnerships (STPs) which themselves will become Integrated Care Systems (ICNs).

3. In New Zealand, with the Ministerial advisory group, commissioned in early 2018, tasked with making recommendations to overhaul the health system, is due to published its interim report in late 2019. Speculation is high that there will be recommendations for structural change, including fewer District Health Boards (DHBs). There is also pressure for the setting up of a standalone National Cancer body.

This article is focused on the fallacy of such structural reforms and some suggestions of a way forward.

Common mistakes

Three common mistakes with most structural reforms are:

1. Not understanding that structures are only one part of an **inter-connected multi-element operating model.**

2. Not focusing on the required changes in mixed of existing and new **talents, capacity, and capability** needed for implementation.

3. Failing to address organization **behaviors, values, and the underlying culture**

Operating Model

The three basics of any structural change agenda are: First, any organization or system structure is part of a multi-element "operating model." High functioning structures are designed to be integrated with other elements of the operating model. Second, creating a specific or target operating model requires plans that provide details of a well-articulated strategy. Third, the strategy itself is developed to deliver on the mission, vision, and purpose. These are the basics that are either glanced over or worst ignored in many reform programs. Any change to operating model will have to test for alignment back to strategy, and checking that the strategies are still relevant.

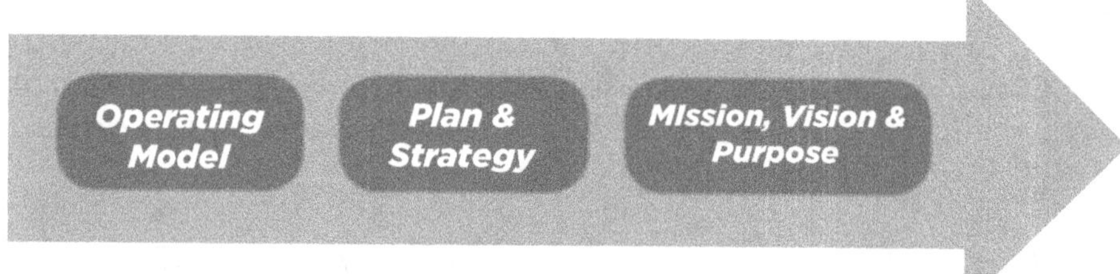

Graphic 1 - The three basics of any structural change agenda

A typical operating model would have the following inter-connected elements.

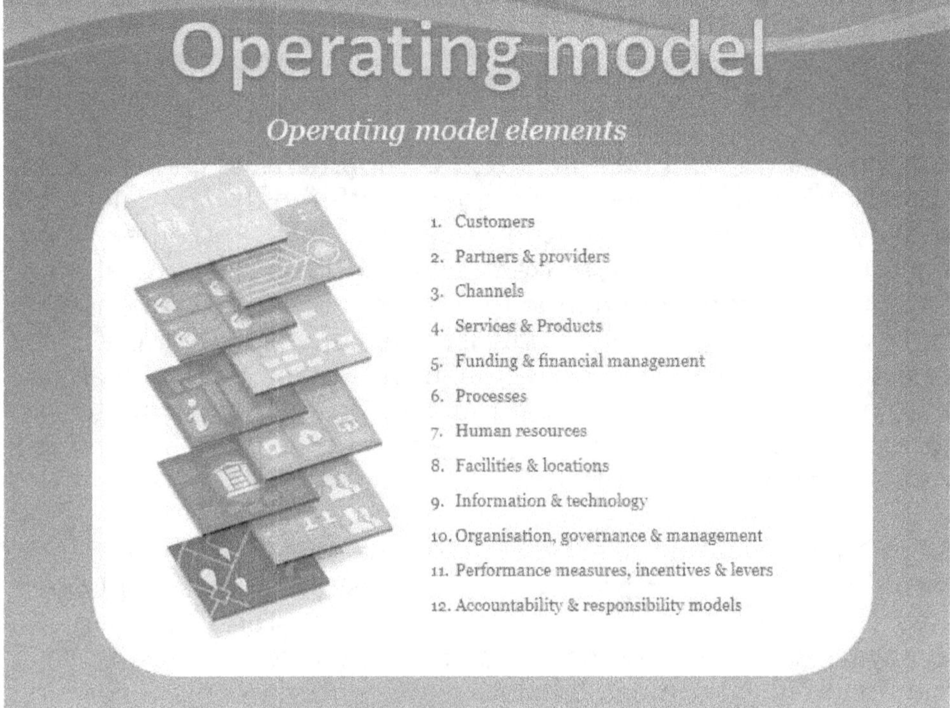

Figure 2 - Operating model elements

The organization, governance, and management layers make up only one of twelve elements. The challenge of any reform agenda is not to tackle any of these elements in isolation. Yet many reform agenda do precisely that! How many times have we seen, a separate "workforce initiative" or "a capital plan for hospital redevelopments" or "an IT ten-year plan."

Suggestion - any change agenda need to pay attention to the three basics as set out above. Undertaking changes to structures should be aligned and integrated with other changes to the elements. Check for connection of the target operating model back to a well-articulated strategy.

Checking that existing strategy is still relevant to fulfill the mission, vision, and purpose, in the light of rapid societal changes. Once the checks are done against the three basics, it should indicate to decision makers that what they are facing is a complex change. Such complex change cannot be executed with just existing talent, capacity, and capability (usually, augmented by management or turnaround consultants).

Talent, capability, and capacity

Implementing a well-designed and comprehensive change to the operating model requires bringing in a different mix of talent, capability, and capacity into the equation. Many implementations stalled because decision makers fail to address this crucial point. One of the reasons for change for current under-performance has to do with existing talent, capability, and capacity. Their practices, knowledge, and skill that once may have worked have been found wanting. Therefore, relying too much on the same people to execute complex system changes is a recipe for failure. This, unfortunately, happens all too often.

Bringing in new talents, capability, and capacity and mixing them with existing high performers ensures fresh thinking without necessary throwing the baby out with the bath water. This mix needs to always start with the senior management team and mid-level management. The most crucial role in ensuring this mix works well as a team rests almost entirely on the shoulder of the Chief Executive. Managing the inevitable tension and clash of ideas between the new and existing needs to done well to make progress. Such tensions are a clear indication of challenges to existing organizational culture, values, and behaviors brought about by the change agenda.

Suggestion - any change agenda requires decision makers to ensure there is a deliberate and right mix of new and existing talents, capability, and capacity. Existing talents, capability, and capability need to those that have demonstrated the ability to have a positive mindset towards the change agenda. Second, pay attention to how tension and managed and mitigated. Not managing such tensions, even if progress could be made, will destroy any trust and relationships needed to establish new cultures, values, and behaviors.

Behaviors, values, and culture

Any changes in healthcare will challenge existing organizational culture, values, and behaviors. The complexity of changes to the multi-elements of an operating is significant and should not be underestimated. Deeply rooted prevailing behaviors, values, and culture lie below the existing process and practices. Therefore, changing them without addressing these underlying behaviors, values, and culture is one of the leading causes of many implementation failures.

The gravitational pull to resist change is always underestimated, and many well thought and funded policies have stalled because changes needed have challenged the beliefs and values of incumbents.

Suggestion - any change agenda requires an early and comprehensive exercise to identify and mitigate gaps between current and desired culture, values, and behaviors. Complex changes require an open, transparent, and no blame culture. There will be a natural resistance to change and having a deliberate process to mitigate and gauge the shift in behaviors, values, and culture throughout any change program is fundamental to embed any early progress.

Final word

Whatever is the structural configuration, centralized or decentralized, it will need all the other elements in the target operating model to be aligned. Any structural configuration when it fails to support better performance and delivers on better health outcome, it does not always mean that the configuration is wrong. The problem may be due to misalignment with other elements of the operating model, or the fault may lie elsewhere in the operating model. Equally, there may be that the issues with existing talents, capacity, and capability, and more importantly, the underlying behaviors, values, and culture itself.

It must not be forgotten that a fundamental assumption in developing and implementing a target operating model, requires plans that provide details of a well-articulated strategy. The strategy itself is designed to deliver on the organization or system mission, vision, and purpose. Without this clear line of sight and alignment between operating model, plans, strategy, mission, vision, and purpose, the risks of any change program, even if successfully executed will deliver something else!

Chapter VI

-

Type And Mix Of Innovations

Is It Important
To Get The Right Type And Mix
Of Innovations To Transform
First World Countries'
Health Systems?

by Chai CHUAH

Following on from my earlier article "Getting serious about making changes in health care?" I want to highlight the importance of understanding the difference between the two types of innovations – sustaining and disruptive.

To meet the complex challenges of First World countries' health systems, both types of innovations are needed. Each type of innovation provides solutions to two common types of complex challenges which are:

1. Improving quality, safety, timeliness, patient experience, efficiency and efficacy for people who can access existing health services.

2. Opening up access to health services in a timely manner for a growing number of people unable to access existing health services. Affordability is normally a major contributing factor.

Some innovative solutions provide answers to (1) while others provide answers to (2). Getting the right type of innovative solutions for the two different type of challenge is fundamental.

It is also important to note that any improvement or innovation agenda needs a portfolio that has the right mix of sustaining and disruptive innovations.

Types of innovation

Innovation involves making products, services or processes better. There are different ways to look at innovations. For the purpose of this article we will stick with how Professor Clayton Christensen classifies innovation.

Sustaining innovations

Sustaining innovations (sometimes referred to as sustaining and efficiency innovations) largely impacts on people who can access existing health services by improving the quality, safety, timeliness, patient experience, efficiency, and efficacy of health services. Exemplars of this type of innovation include well-known health system quality initiative like the SURGICAL CHECKLIST and CHOOSING WISELY.

These initiatives aims to reduce variations, save lives, improve efficiency; reduce waste as well as cost. These in turn provides better care and experience for patients.

The significance of these innovations and improvements is made clear by Dr Atul Gawande in his 2017 interview with Malcolm Gladwell. He observes that lack of proper execution of existing treatments is responsible for over 30% of deaths of people over 75 that can be avoided. This observation is significant given that in most First World countries' over 65s make up on average 15% of the total population and account for 40% to 50% of these countries' total health expenditure.

The Economist March 2nd 2017 article "A digital revolution in health care is speeding up" points out that in rich countries about one-fifth of spending on health care goes to waste, for example on wrong or unnecessary treatments.

Some health leaders argue that there is no more room for "savings" through reducing waste and improving efficiency. However, both Dr Gawande's observation and the Economist article clearly indicate that there is still room for achieving these savings through sustaining innovation improvements.

Disruptive innovations

Disruptive Innovations and improvements open up access to health services in a timely manner for a significant number of people unable to access existing services by making them more affordable.

Disruptive innovation is able to do this by changing health service delivery that involves the use of new technologies supported by new business model that make services more accessible and more affordable. For clarity, service delivery, new technologies and business model are defined as:

· Service delivery involves who, where, when, what and how these services are delivered.

· New technologies are characterised by cheaper and faster

computing power, ubiquitous use of smart phones and other portable devices, digitalisation of information and services making it easier to access, faster to scale and cheaper to develop technology enabled health services. Examples of new technologies includes physical (wearables sensors, robotics, 3D printing of prosthetic and organs), biological (tumbling costs of genome mapping and editing) and advanced digital technologies (AI, Big Data analytics, Cloud based services).

· Business model describes how a service organised its (1) key processes supported by (2) resources to provide a service that provides (3) value to the user in a (4) financially sustainable way.

It is important to invest time to understand the above four elements of a business model. Often in meetings and discussions the term business model is used without a good understanding of what it means.

Some examples of disruptive innovations in health care include:

(1) The CVS Pharmacy is an example of a disruptive innovation in the US pharmacy and primary care sector.
(2) 7 Cups provides free support to people experiencing emotional distress by connecting them with trained listeners.
(3) Mycare helps connect clients and provider in home care, disability support and aged care in New Zealand.
(4) GP at Hand powered by Babylon technology is a new NHS England funded primary care service being trial in a number of locations in England.

Final remarks

Sustaining innovations improve existing services that benefit people already accessing current services. Disruptive innovation opens up affordable access for significant numbers of people missing out on current health services. Both are needed and the challenge is to get the right mix. The two different types of innovations provide solution to two very different problems. That is why it is important to know their differences.

It is important to remember that disruptive innovations involve making changes to both service delivery and all four elements of its business model (value to the user, resources, key processes and sustainable financial formula).

There has always been and most likely always will be resistance to innovations. Some innovations survive while others don't. Professor Calestous Juma in his 2016 book, provides examples of innovations (which we take for granted today) going back 600 years that met significant resistance and survived. He concludes that the underlying reason for this resistance is the disjuncture between rapid technological innovation and the slow pace of institutional adjustment due to a fear of loss. New innovations whether sustaining or disruptive will face the challenge of this disjuncture. Think through the different innovations and improvements in your organisations. Is your organisation got the right innovations for the right problem? I welcome your feedback and comments on this article.

Here are some useful books if you would like to go into greater details some of the material covers in this article.

(1) Seizing The White Space by Mark W. Johnson
(2) The Innovator's Prescription by Clayton Christensen
(3) Innovations and its enemies by Calestous Juma

Likewise here are some YouTube clips referred to in the article:
(1) Professor Clayton Christensen and John Hagel discussion on this important topic of disruptive innovation.
https://www.youtube.com/watch?v=lUmCvHwrPLM&t=1454s

(2)Professor Clayton Christensen explaining the theory behind different types of innovation.
https://www.youtube.com/watch?v=p6vkDm50Bh8&t=1659s

(3) Dr Atul Gawande's interview with Malcolm Gladwell
https://www.youtube.com/watch?v=TKty2axfZxQ&t=1310s

Section-II:
Digital Future and Healthcare

Chapter VII

-

Exponential Technology Driving Change In Healthcare

Slowly, Gradually And Then Suddenly!

by Chai CHUAH

What is this term "exponential technologies" and why is it important to take notice of it?

Let's unpack this. The common example used to explain this term and its impact is the story of a game of chess involving an Indian king and Lord Krishna. The king agreed to grant the deity any reward for beating him. The deity asked for a single grain of rice on the first square and double it on every consequence squares. Having lost the game, every square on the chess board started to be placed with rice as agreed. The king was to have his lesson in the power of exponential growth – 1 grain of rice in square one became over 1,000,000 in the twentieth square and by fortieth first square he was looking at over 1,000,000,000 grains. There are 64 squares on the chess board, you can do the math.

The exponential growth curve starts **_slowly_**, **_gradually_** and then suddenly as the king found out. When the curve reaches the suddenly stage, its impact will be disruptive.

Peter Diamantis and Steven Kotler in their book **_BOLD_** put forward the concept of the 6Ds that is fuelling this exponential growth of today's technologies– digitalization, deception, demonetization, dematerialization, democratization and disruptive.

These technologies are being leveraged by ecommerce digital platform organisations that are led by leaders who have put in place enabling operating, organisation and business models.

What are these digitally enabled ecommerce platform organisations?

Characteristics of these organisations include:
- Their operating, organisation and business models and strategies are underpinned by the 6Ds.
- Their digital platform enables them to scale exponentially.
- Their digital platform also allows them to exit faster and at much lower cost.
- Their digital platform allows them to leverage the power of Big data analytics to understand their customers, operations and develop predictive models.

• Their business interest cross multiple industries, geography and time..
• They use their digital platform to make interactions, transactions and feedback with their consumers and business partners as seamless and effortless as possible.

Amazon, Alibaba, Google and Tencent are some notable examples of such organisations. The last chapter of the book **PLATFORM REVOLUTION** covers "what makes an industry ready for platform revolution?"

The authors highlight certain characteristics that make industries more susceptible to be disrupted by these digital ecommerce platform organisations:

• Information intensive industries
• Industries with non scalable gatekeepers
• High fragmented industries
• Industries characterized by extreme information asymmetries
• Industries with high regulatory control
• Industries with high failure costs
• Resource intensive industries

Healthcare, banking and education industries meet many of the above and yet continue to be resistant to transformative change. The late Professor Calestous Juma in his talk on his latest book, **INNOVATION AND ITS ENEMIES** also identifies healthcare sector as resistant to transformative change.

Exponential technology is going to play centre stage in shaping changes in healthcare. Artificial intelligence, robotics, sensors, blockchain, additive printing, cloud computing, big data analytics, biometric science, new materials, advance genomics sequencing and editing, wearables, autonomous devices, implantables, digestables, virtual/augmented reality are no longer the realms of science frictions and techno geeks. Almost on a daily basis proponents of each of these exponential technologies advocate that their particular flavour of technology is "the one to watch".

The digital nature of all these exponential technologies and their convergence potentially makes it difficult to predict how fast some of them will reach the "suddenly" phase of the exponential curve. What we can be certain is that their digital nature allows them to scale extremely fast within a short space of time and relies on a lower infrastructure investment compared to non digital competitors.

There is a whole digital community out there that is actively working to improve and bring their digital products and services to consumers. Incumbents often underestimated the pace of improvements and potential resulting disruption until it is too late. Following the launch of the refreshed New Zealand Health Strategy in April 2016, a deliberate, difficult but necessary conversation is taking place in the New Zealand health sector.

In the 20 months since this conversation started in New Zealand exponential technologies leveraged by digital enabled ecommerce platform organisations are starting to make their presence felt around the world. The recent Amazon, Berkshire and JP Morgan & Chase announcements, Babylon contracts with NHS England, Google Deepmind and Ping An Good Doctor, are some recent and obvious examples. All of these examples may be well underway towards the "suddenly" part of the exponential curve. Another important question that is often asked is how exponential technology improves patient experience and care.

Increasingly while "experts" debate the efficacy, ethics, privacy and security of these exponential technologies, the practical and sometimes uncomfortable answers lies in how patients and consumers are "subscribing" to these new offerings. Gaps in the 6As - accessible, availability, affordability, appropriateness, awareness and acceptable for patients and consumers being addressed by these exponential technologies becomes the motivating force for change and disruption.

In ten maybe twenty years what will First World countries health system look like? Any answer that looks too much like today is the wrong answer!

Professor Klaus Schwab in his book **"Fourth Industrial Revolution"** issues a warning *"The changes are so profound that, from the perspective of human history there has never been a time of greater promise or potential peril. My concern, however, is that* *decision makers are too often caught in traditional, linear and non disruptive thinking or too absorbed by immediate concerns to think strategically about the forces of disruption and innovation shaping our future"*

So, ultimately finding answers to sustainable future focus health system for First World countries are not just technological challenges it is a leadership one!

In final chapter of his book **Technology versus Technology**, Gerd Leonhard sets out nine principles to guide and fuel this important strategic conversation as well as seven essential questions to ask when evaluating exponential technologies.

 As thought leaders who are interested in this subject matter, this is not a bad place to start our strategic conversations and evaluation of exponential technologies. There is still time but let's not take forever!

Chapter VIII

-

Why Is Healthcare Suddenly Of Interest To Tech Giants?

Like Amazon, Alibaba, Tencent And Samsung

by Chai CHUAH

Towards the end of the 20th century tech giants such as IBM and Microsoft invested in healthcare with mixed success. In the first decade of the 21st century other tech giants like Google and Apple have been increasing their health portfolio investment quietly behind the scenes again with mixed result. Recent news of non-traditional healthcare players making significant investments into health care has stirred up the latest round of interest and discussion in the global healthcare community (at least for those paying attention!).

Examples of those grabbing headlines includes Amazon, Berkshire and JP Morgan joint venture headed by respected global health leader Dr Atul Gawande, the US$ 1 billion acquisition of PillPack by Amazon, a series of announcements by UK based Babylon of new partners (Samsung and Tencent) and launching new AI powered digital health services, recent reported US$1billion plus IPO by the China based Ping An Good Doctor in Hong Kong. There is a sense that the momentum of new entrants disrupting healthcare industry is picking up pace.

Some of the key factors drawing these tech giants into the health care space include:

1. Global health market is conservatively estimated to around US$7 trillion and growing.
2. They are looking at new areas for expansion.
3. Health systems around the world are facing sustainability pressures.
4. Widening unmet needs for health care services presents opportunities.
5. They already provide services to some key determinants of health and well-being - food, retail, recreation, accommodation and transport.
6. New generation of aging baby boomers with resources are prepared to pay for better care and services.
7. They already have connections and relationships with large proportion of population.

Digital platform organisations

What makes these tech giants different from other tech giants of the past? They are ***digital platform organisations***. The most well known are largely Americans (FaceBook, Amazon, Apple, Microsoft and Google, often referred to as FAAMG) and Chinese firms (Alibaba and Tencent). Hot on the heels of these American and Chinese tech giants are other organisations from within their own country such as Baidu, JB Com, Huawei in China, and Netflix, IBM, CISCO, Walmart in the US. Outside of America and China serious contenders includes Softbank (Japan), Samsung (Korea), SAP, Phillips (Europe) and Tata (India). These organisations share certain common features:

1. They either own and/operate a significant digital platform.
2. They investment heavily in cutting edge digital (AI, blockchain, cloud computing), physical (robotics, 3D printing, wearables, new materials) and biological (genomics) technologies.
3. Their digital platform is supported by supercomputing capabilities - processing, storing, analytics and predictive modelling.
4. Their technology architecture enables the fast development of own new applications as well as adoption of other third parties applications.
5. Their technology and business model is design to make it easy and affordable for both consumers and providers of service/products to be part of their network.
6. Their technology and business model enables rapid adoption, modifying, scaling, and downsizing.
7. They are driven by creating value for their network users (both consumers and providers of services/products).
8. They augment their physical services with digital online services that allow them to operate across time zones and geographical locations.
9. Data and the interactions between their users are the fuel for their business model to create value.
10. They have diverse industries portfolio and are main investors behind young unicorn start-ups globally.

Not too long ago these tech giants pretty much stick to their respective ecommerce, social media, messaging, search engine, smart devices and consumer products markets. The very nature of their platform business models however requires them to constantly look at providing more services to their users. This has resulted in two key movements:

1. Their entry into new services such as cloud computing, banking, insurance, share riding, robotics and wearables.

2. Crossing over into each other's traditional markets.

Disruption to industries

Globally, these tech giants have disrupted a number of industries including taxis, accommodations, retail, music, publishing, photography, logistics, manufacturing, and IT services. To-date there remains a number of industries that have not been significantly disrupted by these tech giants. These include healthcare, banking, insurance, education, construction & infrastructure redevelopment, housing, energy, transport (sea, air, rail and road), food supply and production and professional services (accounting, legal, architecture and engineering). These will be the new markets for these tech giants. Some incumbents in these industries are making serious efforts to transition to either collaborate or compete with these new entrants.

The jury is still out whether these incumbents can make the transition. To succeed they have to overcome a number of big factors:

1. speed of decision making,

2. appetite for new ideas,

3. quantum of investment,

4. taking a long term view and

5. ability to absorb short term set-backs

These tech giants knocking on their front door are prepared to make quick decisions and comfortable to operating in a fast and constantly changing environment. The size of their investments is staggering and the diversity of their investments is breath-taking. Case in point is the current investment portfolio of the much publicised US$100 billion SoftBank Vision Fund that includes biotechnology, insurance, construction, ecommerce, property, semiconductors, agrotechnology, digital mapping, self driving cars, robotics software, data infrastructure, healthcare and online payments and virtual reality.

https://www.economist.com/leaders/2018/05/12/the-meaning-of-the-vision-fund

Entry into healthcare

These new players will bring with them a whole suite of new and converging technologies that will push a number of boundaries in healthcare services. They will also bring with them insights, lessons learnt and expertise developed from their diverse portfolio. Early targets will be in any health services where data can be digitalised, AI and machine learning applications developed such as in early screening, assessment, monitoring, diagnostics and certain treatment therapies. This will change the landscape of self-care, home-care, community care, residential care, primary care and hospital care in the next 5 to 10 years.

As these new entrants make their entry into health care they will and are finding at this stage a "challenging and difficult" reception from incumbents. This is nothing new to them. New entrants are more likely to make progress quickly at the "edges" where the incumbents have fleeting interest or have run out of new ideas of what to do. Conversely, new entrants trying to enter into the core services of the incumbents are unlikely to make progress for the simple reason that in the core services incumbents' vested interest, influence and power are strongest.

So where can we find the current edges in health care – this will be where there is the significant unmet need and where there is the greatest dissatisfaction amongst current users of health services. Mental health services, access to primary care, access to elective treatment and anything to do with non-acute services for seniors. Partners for these tech giants

For these tech giants to succeed in healthcare they will need to find health leaders and organisations to partner with. Tech giants will be looking for health care partners that these tech giants that share their vision, appetite for change and ability to harness the potential of new technologies.

The millennials working in healthcare are obvious candidates but there are others. That is why the appointment of Dr. Atul Gawande as CEO of the new Amazon, Berkshire and JP Morgan health venture is such a master stroke. Recent events unfolding in NHS England with movements to accelerate the adoption of a digital first primary care service model is also very encouraging.

Final word

Many challenges lie ahead for these tech giants and their health partners. No doubt not everything they try in the healthcare space will work and there be some dead-ends, detours and pausing. There is no doubt and the data points of their interest in health care are clear. They are here to stay.

The recent reported quote by Jeff Bezos on their new health venture is worth noting "***we said at the outset that the degree of difficulty is high and success is going to require an expert's knowledge, a beginner's mind and a long term orientation***". What works in their favour is that they understand the importance of needing to constantly add value to the changing needs of their users. To the incumbents and decision makers in healthcare industry (clinicians, politicians, policy makers, health funders and providers, board members, Chief Executives and union leaders) ready or not you have new company – the tech giants!

Chapter IX

-

Health Systems Pressure Can Only Be Solved By Addressing Social Determinants

by Chai CHUAH

In my previous chapters, makes the point that doing more of the same will not provide solutions to ongoing and growing pressures of health services. This article covers the need to address social determinants if we are serious about finding answers to relief health system pressure.

The World Health Organisation published a report in 2008 entitled "Closing the gap in a generation: health equity through action on the social determinants of health. Final Report of the Commission on Social Determinants of Health". More than ten years on it remains a very useful resource to guide policies and actions on social determinants.

Social determinants have always been a significant driver of healthcare need. However, despite greater awareness and urgency to address social determinants, progress in addressing these determinants to-date has been too slow. The consequences have now caught up with many First world countries as evidenced by increased social issues such as increased poverty, homelessness, family violence, substance abuse, food banks, anxiety, and depression. On a positive note, some of the more enlightened health leaders and organizations are taking steps to address their patient's and community's social needs as well as their health needs.

Such actions, although commendable and beneficial to individuals receiving such support, add a more significant burden on health systems that are already under pressure. But it does not address the conditions or determinants that created these social needs. Addressing social needs without addressing the determinants that caused them is yet another ambulance at the bottom of the cliff.

Social needs versus social determinants

The January 2019 article in Health Affairs draws out the difference between social determinants and social needs. This article explains the difference between the two.

Social determinants, as pointed out in this article, is defined as "conditions in which people are born, grow, live, work, and age" and "the fundamental drivers of these conditions." The focus is a broad, community-wide focus on the underlying social and economic conditions in which people live, rather than the immediate needs of any one individual.

By contrast, social needs, especially in the context of driving health services, are defined by accommodation, food, transport, welfare and income support of individuals recovering from illness or living with chronic health conditions. The lack of access to these basic needs directly impacts on the individual's ability to get well, stay well, and live a healthy life.

Unfortunately, while addressing social needs benefits individuals, it is yet another ambulance at the bottom of the cliff scenario since the deficiencies in the underlying social determinants remain unresolved.

Addressing these underlying social determinants deficiencies requires both a transformative policy program and a different implementation capability.

Policy

Government (local, regional, national and international) are primarily responsible for policies that create conditions and environment for its citizens to be born, work, play, live, raise their families, age and contribute to society.

Social need comes about when social determinants policies lag too far behind changes in societal values, practices, and expectations. The extent of the social need is a direct result of the gap between societal values, traditions, expectations, and social determinants — the more significant the gap, the higher demand for social need, and vice versa.

Many countries in recent times, faced with the exponential rate of change in societal values, beliefs, and practices have struggled to come up with much needed timely policy responses. For example, smaller family size, urban drift, longer life expectancy, demographic changes, growing income gaps, and changes in lifestyle, have stretched, disrupted, and ultimately strained existing social and economic systems.

Likewise, increasing and significant natural disasters, as well as war and conflicts, have led to catastrophic humanitarian emergencies and global movement of refugees and migrants, further magnifying social determinants deficiencies.

These complex set of drivers have created overwhelming social needs that will frustrate even the very best of efforts by health services to contribute to the population's well-being.

In many countries, pre-21st-century political ideology, and futile theatre of politics makes it difficult for the government to provide policy leadership.

A transformative policy agenda can only come from future-focused and courageous political leaders supported by public services institutions that need to unshackle themselves from pre-21st-century mindset and capabilities.

Implementation

The above WHO report is a useful resource that tells readers "what" constitute social determinants with recommendations on "what" actions are needed. It does not and cannot provide answers to "how." It is the "how" to implement a transformative policy program that to-date has eluded many First world countries. Implementation of a comprehensive policy program requires a diverse group of non-government stakeholders such as private sectors, professional groups, unions, academia, community" and civil society. With such a diverse group of participants, one the immediate challenge is to manage competing agendas and vested interests. Overcoming this challenge requires a new mindset, capability, capacity, and talent that can grapple with the complexity of implementing a transformative policy program.

Final word

The work on addressing social determinants to this day remains a work in progress, and the demand to address social needs will continue to grow. Health systems are now having to step into the space of addressing social needs, which will add further pressure on the health systems. Health systems involvement in addressing social needs is still a version of an ambulance at the bottom of the cliff. For now, it is a necessary part of the transition to provide more comprehensive support for those in greatest need. But it is unsustainable. Those wishing to address and relief the pressures on the health system need to go further upstream into the realms of addressing social determinants. Of late there have been some new entrants into health system from outside of health. Some bring with them a platform approach that offers the opportunity to put social determinants firmly on their platform agenda.

The dual challenge of a developing transformative policy program and a disciplined implementation to strengthen social determinants is possible. An example is the 2017 landmark implementation of pay equity policy with a budget of NZ$2 billion to increase the pay for 55,000 low paid mainly female dominated home and residential support workers in the New Zealand health and disability sector. This example demonstrates that it is possible to implement a transformative policy in 10 weeks after legislative approval!

In the exponential curve of interventions to relieve pressures on the health system, addressing social needs is a positive, necessary but still insufficient. Relief will only come from making positive changes to current social determinants.

Chapter X

-

Winter Pressure & Call For More Funding

by Chai CHUAH

Whenever First World countries health system comes under pressure such as England in this recent winter there is the inevitable call for "more investment into health services". As the southern hemisphere prepares for their winter demand will it end up with the same predictable result of "the system cannot cope and on the brink of health service failure and more funding is needed".
This call for more investment has some justification when First World countries faces

• Increasing demand pressure driven by ageing population, people living longer (often with more years in poor health), increasing burden of complex life long, lifestyle related ill health and greater expectations from society, and

•   Increasing supply pressure in the form of ageing workforce, higher cost of drugs and technology and the need to invest in additional and more modern facilities.

Most First World countries that have increased funding have in one form or another also reviewed related issues of effectiveness of their funding and/or the sustainability of their current funding policies. Such reviews will touch on the broader issue of wastage, efficiency and efficacy of existing funding in health services such as:

• How funding are allocated to delivery organizations
• What and how current health programme are being commissioned,
• More investment into more hospital beds, rest and nursing home beds, respite beds, primary care, home and social support services
• More investment into workforce and IT systems
• More investment into research and increase publicly funded "personalized medicines and therapies".

Despite reform efforts on the above there is no relief in sight for pressures on First World countries health systems. Why?

Funding on its own not enough to address the pressure

Because funding althoughan important ingredient is only one element of a health eco-system. More funding without changing other fundamentals of the health eco-system will not address the pressure but could actually be making it worst by delaying the need for a more comprehensive and substantive reform.

Other fundamentals such as models of care, enabling policies, regulations, accountability and performance levers, organization structures, business models and other enablers (workforce, technology, facilities, advance Big Data analytics, devices, etc) need to be part of a total package of reform to address the sustainability question.

Too often reforms are either fragmented or done in isolation, example setting up a separate "advisory group" for workforce, organization structures, infrastructure or technology, etc. Even when an overarching "whole of system advisory group" is commissioned, recommendations on these fundamentals are design to optimize each of the individual elements rather than the whole system.

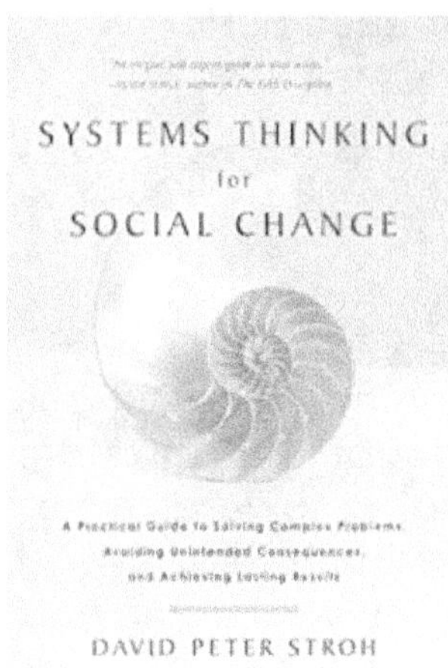

System thinking

System thinking is a pre-requisite for making real and sustainable changes to social services like health services. The author David Stroh in his 2015 book "System thinking for social change" provides a practical guide to solve complex social problems, avoiding unintended consequences and achieving lasting results. There are some very challenging chapters that clearly indicates that what is being done currently is actually making the situation worst not better.

Leadership and talent

Taking a system approach to change these fundamentals requires a different level of leadership and talent to the ones that manages these fundamentals. The mindset, process, skill, knowledge and experience of leaders who manages the system versus those who will change it is not the same. Most current health leaders are there to manage the current system and will often take the position that "more money, resources and time" are needed. Most struggle with the current let alone being asked to do something about the future.

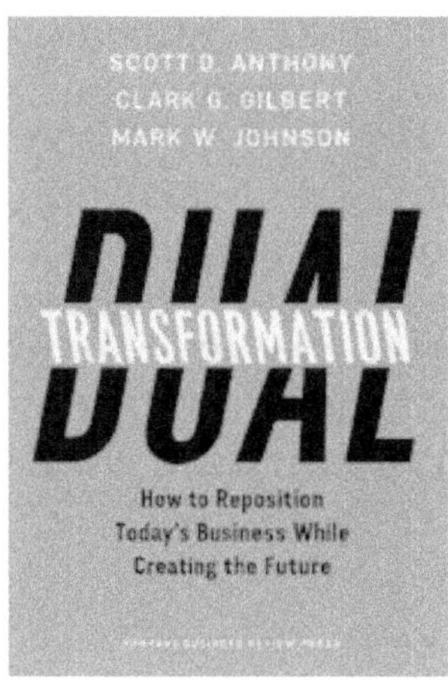

Dual transformation

We need leaders that can handle the pressure of managing the current system with a bias to creating a new system – a dual transformation endeavor. The authors Scott Antony, Clark Gilbert, Mark Johnson in their 2017 book "Dual Transformation" provides useful insights into what it takes to manage today's business while creating the future. The A, B and C concept requires different leadership and talent for each part.

Concluding remarks

The health system is big expenditure with significant social impact in any First World country. There is no doubt that the tidal wave of pressure feels unmanageable and heading towards a tipping point. Funding on its own is not enough. Each First World country should critically look at whether it has the leadership and talent it needs to take on a dual transformation approach to start to change course towards a more sustainable system. Otherwise every year it will face the inevitable chorus of "more funding is needed". *If you read this article and having a go at creating the leadership and talent for the dual transformation I am interested to hear from you.*

Chapter XI

-

Art or Science? Financial Management Of Health System

by Chai CHUAH

Running to stand still: Why £20.5bn is a lot but not enough to do everything

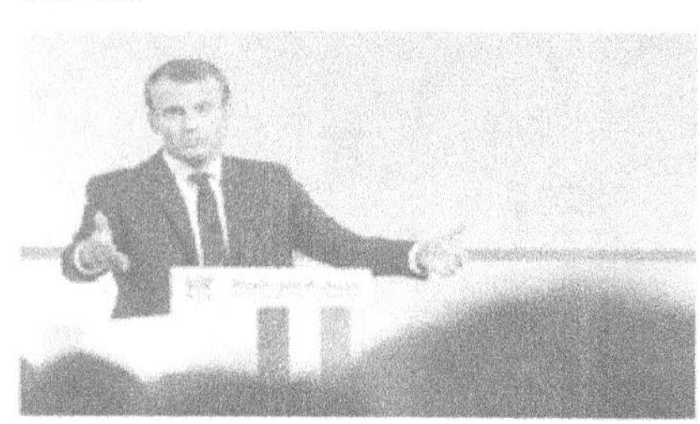

Macron announces changes to France's health care system

Underfunding of health system leads to $240m blowout - Health Minister

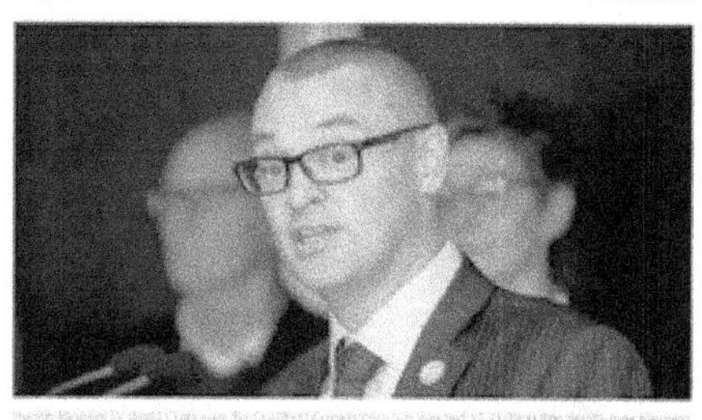

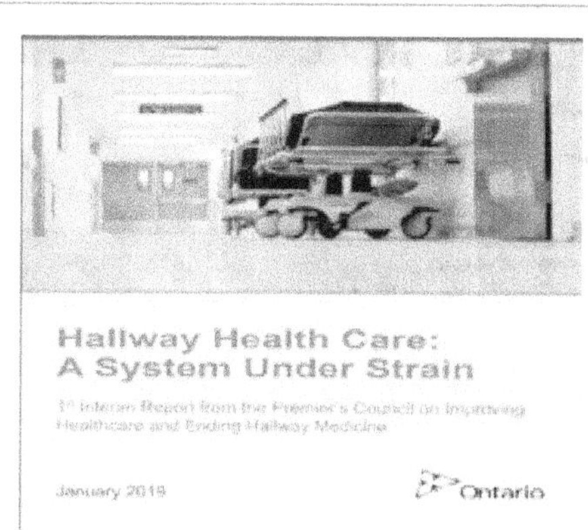

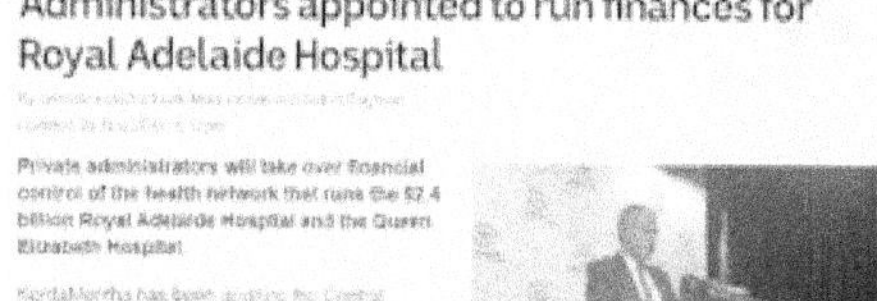

Administrators appointed to run finances for Royal Adelaide Hospital

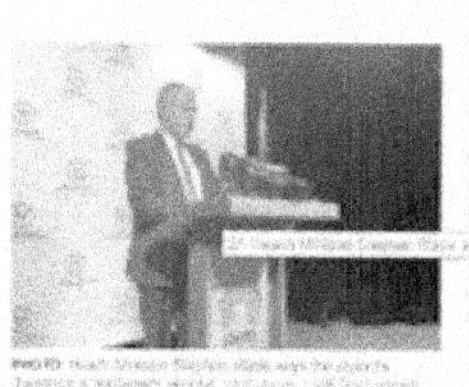

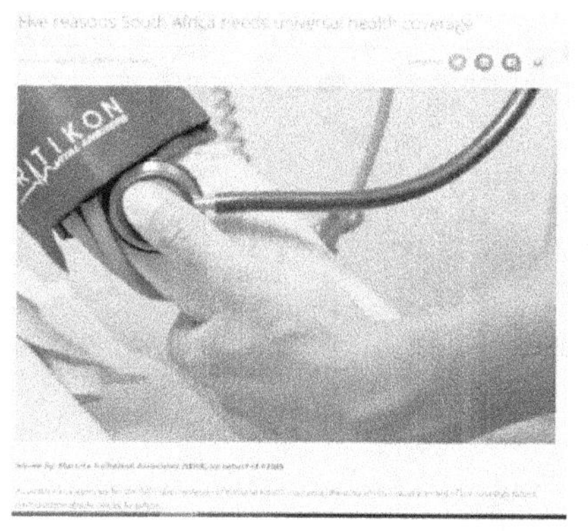

Context

With growing and aging population, it is not unreasonable to expect more investment into healthcare. The well-being and health of a population is of course influenced by other determinants that are equally important. It is pointless just throwing more funding to solve health system pressures without addressing these other determinants.

It is also a duty and responsibility of those running health system to be good fiscal stewards of funding received. The evidence to-date would suggest that it is easier said than done.

In the second half of 2018, articles from a number of First world countries health system reported their health system under financial pressure. France, Australian States, Canadian Provinces, New Zealand, South Africa and NHS England1 are in various stages of downward financial spiral.

Those responsible for the system (politicians, clinicians, and managers) and other commentators blame "years of under-funding" as one the main reasons for the current financial state. Governments are in various stages of seeking advice and undertaking "expert" reviews looking for answers.

Recommendations are likely to include for more and different types of funding, for more resources to deliver more services, some form of structural reforms, better integration with social care, introduce or re-introduce funder/provider split, user-pay and some form of new or enhance universal health insurance. In more recent times other recommendations now include better use of "Big Data" and faster adoption of digital, physical and biological technologies. Many of these recommendations frequently come with the caveat that more funding is needed for such changes to become a reality.

Implementation of such reforms also needs a relook at financial management. Current fiscal deficits are partly due to a failure of financial management. The financial management system in healthcare needs an overhaul; otherwise, it could frustrate future health system's reforms and transformation.

This paper looks at some salient aspects of financial management in the health system.

A Story to Start With

In my first lecture of accounting in my first undergraduate year, the lecturer explained why accounting is the oldest profession in the world. He said that in the Bible, that before God created the world, there was chaos! He said who do you think created the chaos? The accountant of course!

While it is only a story, behind every financial crisis will be the "accountant" who help keep the records as the disaster unfolded. Of course, there are many noble, civic-minded and talented accountants in every sector and industries including healthcare doing a perfectly good job. So, what's going on in almost all First world countries health system facing a significant financial crisis that threatens to spiral out of control and where are the gaps in financial management?

As a chartered accountant, I started my career in an international accounting and management consulting firm. Thirty-eight years later I finished my career as the Director-General of Health and Chief Executive of the New Zealand Ministry of Health. The comments below reflect my experience in healthcare over the last 27 years.

Financial Management In Healthcare

Financial management of health systems is both an art and a science. The science is the various smart funding, accounting, and financing technique to record revenue and expenditure. The art has two parts. The easy part is to ensure financial records reflects why, who, what, where and how clinical services are delivered. The hard part is to support the complex challenge of making changes to clinical and health services.

This article highlights key aspects of financial management that health system leaders should understand at any time not when they are facing financial pressure.

Accounting Policies Affecting Operating Results

Accounting policies such as depreciation, amortisation, revaluation, capitalisation of expenses, revenue recognition rules, accruals, and provisions can have a significant impact on the operating results of health organisations.

The recording of expenses needs to reflect the reality of resource utilisation operationally. Likewise, the recording of revenue needs to reflect the reality of work done in accordance with agreed funding contracts.

It is critically important when significant deficits are reported that separating out the impact of one-off or recurring expenses and revenue from operational realities is crucial. Clarity is important to understand the impact on financial performance as a result of operational decisions versus those driven by accounting policies.

While clinical leaders and most operational managers are not be expected to understand such accounting nuances, it is important that other decision makers at management and governance level ensure that such decisions on accounting policies are appropriate.

Funding Need To Support Delivery Of Health Outcomes

The design, implementation, monitoring, and management of funding needs to be based on what services are needed to deliver health outcomes that address the health needs of the population. There are multiple types of health services needed to look after a population's health ranging from health promotion, prevention, screening, early intervention, primary, hospital, palliative, and end-of-life care. Clinical and health services can be straight forward and simple, while others are complicated or complex.

Different processes and resources are needed to deliver these very different simple, complicated and complex services. Therefore, funding methods need to likewise reflect such differences. Different methods of funding health services such as fee for service (FFS), price volume capped funding, bulk population funding and service development funding need to be applied appropriately to these three different categories of services.

FFS funding is appropriate for simple and straight forward services, where the health needs are well defined, the intervention and the outcome required are both clear. This funding arrangement is most appropriate for elective services. Performance metrics measuring the number of health services delivered (e.g. the number of elective surgeries on major joints) and specific health outcome (e.g. return to work) are needed to accompany metrics on volume of service delivered.

Price volume capped funding with a flexibility margin for unders and overs may be appropriate for complicated services. This funding arrangement is suitable for acute services where demand is unpredictable. Performance metrics focus on the impact on specific health outcome (e.g. reduce the level of patients dying while on the waiting list) and volume of services delivered (number of patients treated).

Bulk population-based funding is appropriate when health needs and outcomes require a portfolio of interventions ranging from prevention, early treatment, monitoring, and management. This funding arrangement is suitable for complex chronic conditions requiring a portfolio of programmes ranging from prevention, screening, early intervention, and palliative care aimed at chronic, lifelong and lifestyle conditions rather than episodic events. Performance metrics measuring the impact of the portfolio of activities on health needs and health outcome tend to be more complex. The focus is not how measuring how successful in each siloed activity but the relationship and collective impact on the population health needs and outcomes.

Service development funding is appropriate to support the establishment of a new service or substantial expansion of an existing service. The outcome for such a funding method is the establishment of a service capability. The performance metrics will tend to focus on achieving a milestone for recruiting staff, setting up IT and other systems as well as facilities. Performance metrics focus on setting up of key operational processes and putting place human and other key resources within an agreed timeframe. Service development funding needs to have a clear pathway to an ongoing service delivery funding (either FFS or bulk).

Expenditure Management

Traditionally, when health system comes under financial pressure, one of the remedial actions will be to look at tightening up its baseline expenditure.

An assumption is made that there are wastage, inefficiency, and lack of productivity in the health system. As a principle, this is not an unreasonable position to take. However, such an assumption needs to be based on a higher principle - a health system that will provide more accessible, equitable, effective, efficient, high quality and sustainable services that will improve the health and well-being of its population.

The science of traditional expenditure management at a time of financial pressure is textbook. The prescription will include:

1. Managing staff costs – staff numbers, remuneration levels, entitlements,

2. Managing consumables – prices, range of choices, level of inventory, contractual and procurement terms,

3. Managing facilities costs – reducing the number of locations, smaller facilities, deferring repairs, and maintenances,

4. Managing new programmes – deferring, reducing the scope and reducing resources needed,

5. Changing accounting policies – capitalising operating expenses, extending the useful life of assets, revising downwards recognition of future liabilities, deferring write-off of obsolete assets,

The problem with the above approach, it does not address the real underlying reasons for the financial pressures – health services models not able to keep up with demand.

Financial and non-financial performance metrics

Financial performance metrics first and foremost need to provide insight into how services are organised and executed operationally. Such insights can only be gain by looking at both financial and non-financial performance metrics.
Better insights can be gained when looking at appropriate operational and financial metrics together.

Operational decisions in service delivery drive activities that consume resources. For financial reports to be meaningful it has to read alongside operational metrics that measure resources consumed, activities performance, outputs produced and outcomes achieved.

Performance metrics - too much, too little, Questions & decisions

Performance metrics need to achieve a dual purpose – to understand what happened in the past to inform current decisions.

Performance metrics provides the starting point to ask questions and make sense of the answers to gauge how clinical and managers manage their services throughout the month. Too much information can make it difficult to make sense of different insights. Positive and negative financial variances against budget are meaningless unless they are considered alongside non-financial metrics. For example, a positive expenditure variance could mean that the planned service activities have not been delivered. Conversely, a negative expenditure variance with a significant over-delivery against planned service activities should invite discussion on what is driving the increased level of activities.

Discussions on positive or negative deviations from plans provide a window into the planning process and the operational reality. The ultimate goal of any performance metrics is to make decisions today using performance metrics insights to impact the future. High performing health leaders produce meaningful reports to provide insights for appropriate actions to improve service and ultimately organisation performance.

Better insights from trends

Performance metrics that focus on the comparison of actuals against budgets or last year actuals need to be complemented by looking at trends of actuals. Looking at the trend of both actual financial and non-financial metrics provides a different insight from just the variance against the budget. Such insights into how fast or slow changes are occurring can open up different discussions on what is happening to clinical services and actions required.

Need more than a "one size fits all" Performance metrics

Health organisation needs to constantly innovate to be sustainable and relevant in an exponentially changing environment and context. Professor Clayton Christensen2, an internationally recognised thought leader and the author points out that organisations need to have a balanced portfolio of three types of innovation -" efficiency, sustaining and market-creating".

Both efficiency and sustaining innovations focus on improving processes to deliver more cost-effective existing services to existing users. It does not make existing services available to those who are missing out. Market-creating innovations develop services that open up affordable access to those currently unable to access existing services.

Different financial performance metrics are needed to support the three different types of service innovations. A one size fits all financial performance metrics is not appropriate for organisations with a mixed portfolio of service delivery and innovations.

For example, financial metrics such as RONA and IRR for these three very different types of innovations need to be different. However, in many organisations the same financial metrics are used to gauge the success or otherwise of these three types of investments.

Many organisations financial metrics tend to focus on "efficiency" activities rather than the other two. As a result, business case and proposal for "creating new markets" activities struggle to get support. Without creating new markets and solely focusing on efficiency or even sustaining innovations is the main reason why many health organisations are facing service and financial pressures. In such organisations, financial performance metrics are part of the problem.

Costings

Costing exercises will need to be carried out periodically to understand cost movements and often used to inform discussions on prices and funding levels. Such costing exercise will make assumptions on:

- resource requirements to directly provide the service,
- allocation of service, facility and organisation overheads.
- efficiency, effectiveness, and productivity

The judgment rendered on the last two assumptions requires senior financial leaders' oversight in consultation with clinical and service management leaders. Many of the service, facility, and organisation overheads are fixed and the allocation method needs to support the strategic intent of the service, facility, and organisation. Efficiency, effectiveness and productivity assumptions need to informed by the commitment and ability of clinicians and service managers to execute.

Costing exercise will often provide information on significant variations between the original baseline prices and the revised costs for different services. Any such adjustments if carried out should be made for all services rather than cherry picking on some services showing huge variations between reworked cost and original prices. This needs to be a strategic decision rather just a technical decision as any significant changes in prices are often the subject of much debate between the providers and the funders.

Preparing budgets

Preparing the budget of health institution is a complex exercise. The challenge is to ensure that financial budgets are informed by how clinical leaders and managers plan to provide the service.

Setting both the annual and monthly budgets need to come from discussions with clinical leaders and managers. They need to provide insights into how they plan to deliver the service. Phasing of budgets using last years actual or multi-year trends are valid provided it reflects how services will be delivered in the coming year. With the best of intention, it is likely that actual delivery of services will be different from what has been budgeted. Positive and negative variance of actuals of financial non-financial metrics is prima facie neither good or bad. It invites the reader to ask questions to get an understanding of how services were delivered and managed during the month.

Budgeting for clinical services should be at a departmental level. Departments budgets can be prepared as a "cost centre" rather than "profit centre". The author recommends that a cost centre approach is preferred for the reasons outlined below. Costs to be budgeted should be on "controllable direct cost" to deliver the required volume of different services provided by the department.

The budgeting of organisation overheads should be done at an organisation level rather than be allocated and budgeted at a department level. There are two main reasons for this approach. First, such overheads are not controllable by clinical service departments, and secondly, allocation to departments almost inevitably leads to unproductive discussions on the fairness of allocations.

The final budget of the organisation will need to show how the organisation intends to manage its direct controllable costs as well as its overheads within the funding it receives to deliver the required level of services. Budgets should be finalised before a financial year starts and the process of finalising the budgets will require several iterations. The challenge is to have a final budget that achievable with enough flexibility to challenge departments to look at delivering efficient, effective and productive services.

Cost centre or profit centre

How health organisations hold their various services to account for performance matters. Services can be structured as a cost centre or profit centre. Both are technically valid ways to organise services for accountability. However, there are broad implications that go beyond a simple "accounting" matter.

Cost centre services are design to focus on how they manage their cost in delivering their services. Profit centre services are designed to focus on the "bottom-line profit". Both drives very different behaviors that may or may not be helpful depending on how health systems are funded.

A profit centre approach requires allocation of revenue for services delivered, transfer pricing of work done by supporting departments, and allocation of indirect costs and organisation overheads. The focus is whether the clinical services are profitable. While this is a valid financial management technique, it brings with it a lot of "accounting" work that requires resources. Organisations who follows a profit centre approach will encounter a lot more discussions and debate on the fairness of revenue allocation, transfer pricing, allocation of indirect costs and organisation overheads. A profit centre approach brings with it eventually a culture of competition between departments.

Under a cost centre approach, a clinical service department is given a cost budget to deliver an agreed level of service. One version of cost centre approach focuses only on getting clinical service departments to be accountable for their "controllable direct costs". This approach required clinical leaders and managers to manage resources that directly relates to service delivery. Fixed, indirect costs and organisation overhead costs are also managed as cost centres. Revenue budgets under a cost centre approach are normally held at a facility or organisation level. The objective under a cost centre approach is to focus on ensuring that the organisation has budgeted sufficient resources to deliver services within the overall revenue provided to the organisation.

Capital expenditure

In today's environment when technology and science are changing at a rapid pace, inappropriate capital expenditure decisions can "lock" organisations to health services delivery practices long past their use-by dates.

Capital expenditure and their impact on operating expenditure often can be the leading cause of financial problems of health organisations. Investments in facilities and technology are significant investments in healthcare. Most health organisations when it comes to capital expenditure are confronted with two deficits:

1. a weak balance sheet that cannot support investments in significant capital expenditure without equity contributions and/or borrowings.

2. lack of governance, clinical and management expertise to manage large capital projects.

Many health organisations struggle to properly manage the implementation of big capital projects. Most health organisations do not recognise the need for dedicated governance and project leadership with appropriate subject matter experts on specific capital expenditure types. Clinical input supported by other experts, sound change management, good communication, and skillful programme management is vital ingredients to prevent delays and cost blow-outs.

Managing all 3 financial statements

Sound financial management requires an oversight over the "3 financial statements" – Operating Statement, Balance Sheet and the Cashflow Statement. The insights from looking at the inter-relationship of information presented in these three documents provide a more complete picture of the financial affairs of any organisation.

Too many health organisations focus too much on just the Operating Statement at the expense of the other two documents. For example, a sudden increase in "assets" may indicate deferral of operating expenses. Similarly, an increase in provisions of liabilities could explain sudden increases in costs (especially at year-end).

Watching cashflow is essential especially for organisations with operating deficits. Early cashflow problems can often be "hidden" by deferring paying expenses or getting advances of funding. Both these examples can quickly be picked up by paying attention to the Balance Sheet movements.

Most governance board will have a "Finance and Audit" committee that need to provide oversight over the movements of these three financial statements. Health organisations in financial deficits indicate a weakness in this crucial governance oversight.

Forecasting

Preparing short, medium or long-range forecast can either be helpful or a hindrance in health care. Most forecasts bear little resemblance to reality because of flawed assumptions. The challenge with a medium and long-range forecast in healthcare is anticipating the impact of exponential changes in demand. The preparation of the forecast should come out of a broader strategic exercise by an organisation to look out into the future.

A forecast prepared on the assumptions that current services and models of delivery will remain unchanged can be useful to provide a "counter-factual" future scenario. This scenario is more than likely to show the need for very significant funding for both operating and capital expenditures.

A second and different forecast is required. This scenario can start with the counter-factual with changes to incorporate efficiency, sustaining and disruptive innovations. This second forecast needs to have a low, medium and high version to reflect the uncertainty of such an exercise.

Both scenarios of forecasts provide decision makers of a picture of what the future could look like under different assumptions. The forecast should be prepared and looked at as a minimum on a quarterly basis.

Conclusion

Financial management in health organisations is part of a broader complex management system. The science part is the latest technique, standards, tools, and frameworks. The art part is choosing the right "science" to inform and support the delivery of health services. The subject matter covered above is by no means an exhaustive list of topics to consider in managing the finances of health organisations. It is, however, the basics that need to be done well.

References

1. South Australian health network under financial administration. ***https://www. abc.net.au/news/2018-11-26/administrators-appointed-to-run-adelaide-lo- cal-health-network/10554996.***

2. NHS hospitals is sliding into increasing deficits. ***https://www.kingsfund.org. uk/projects/nhs-in-a-nutshell/trusts-deficit.***

3. NZ hospitals increasing financial deficits. ***https://www.nzherald.co.nz/nz/ news/article.cfm?c_id=1&objectid=12133330.***

4. French health system under financial pressure. ***https://www.reuters.com/ar- ticle/us-france-health/macron-injects-cash-to-fix-frances-healthcare-system- idUSKCN1LY1L8***

5. Professor Clayton Christensen 2017 presentation. ***https://www.youtube.com/ watch?v=lUmCvHwrPLM***

Chapter XII

-

Better Health Outcomes, Reducing Inequities And Balancing The Books

Is It No Longer Possible?

by Chai CHUAH

I recently completed an online four-part course called Future Learn, run by the King's Fund. I thoroughly enjoyed this online learning course. The business model starts with free participation, and for a small fee participant get an "upgrade." Of course, I upgraded! Well done King's Fund.

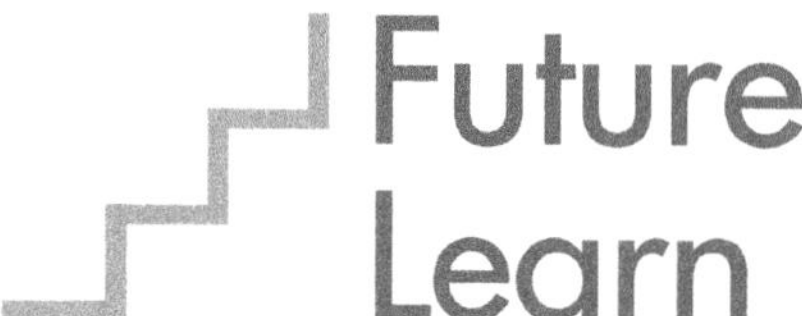

In week 3, part of the content covered important issues of "better outcomes, reducing inequalities and balancing the books." The question is **"Should the NHS prioritize <u>patient outcomes</u> above <u>financial performance</u>, access and addressing <u>health inequalities</u>?"** For this article I have replaced inequalities with inequities. While inequality is important the real issue for many health systems is inequity.

Increasingly, those responsible for managing today's health systems are retreating from the idea that achieving all three objectives is not possible and trade-offs between them are becoming the norm.

How did we get to this point?

The graph below provides a useful insight into how we got to this point.

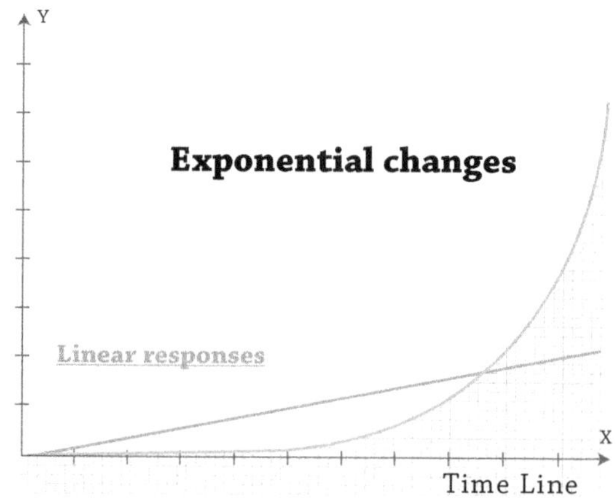

Graphic 2 - Insight into exponential changes

In simple terms, it is the story of changes in demand and supply moving at a different pace. Changes in demand are moving along on the **exponential curve** while health system supply responses continue to change on the **linear line.**

The narrative of this graph has two parts:

Part 1 - where supply responses exceeded demand expectations. Advances in public health, prevention programmes, the introduction of new diagnostic and screening programmes, the breakthrough in new therapeutic medicine and novel treatment techniques throughout the 20th century has been a significant reason for increasing human life expectancy.

Part 2 - where demand has exceeded supply. This is today's 21st-century reality for many First world health systems. This growing chasm is the domain of widening inequities, growing fiscal deficits, uneven and potentially poor health outcomes.

Demand-side changes, moving on an exponential curve trajectory driven by the speed, volume, frequency, and convergence include:

1. Demographic and social changes
2. Environmental (physical and climatic) changes
3. Scientific, engineering and technology changes
4. Political and economic changes

The complexity, uncertainty, and ambiguity of these changes make it challenging to respond traditionally. The consequence and impact on individuals, families, communities, and population have become difficult to predict. The recent forest fires in California with its devastating impact is a case in point.

Many of these changes in its early stages to the casual observer look very benign and inconsequential. However, its exponential trajectory will accelerate to a "J" or "hockey stick" point. When that happens demand changes will quickly catch up with any slag in the supply line, cross the "tipping point" before racing ahead and opening up the gap between the two.

Stephen Kotler's concept of 6Ds (digitalization, democratization, demonetization, deception, and disruption) provides one of the better explanations on why the exponential curve behaves this way. The book BOLD by Stephen and Peter Diamandis goes into some depth to explain the impact of the 6Ds.

Supply responses contributing to this gap include:

1. Discovery, trials, development, adoption cycle takes too long and too expensive.
2. Fixed and static facilities dominate health service delivery practices.
3. Cottage industry or industrial era practices dominants health service delivery, organization, business, and management models.
4. Workforce training and development emphasized specialization, takes a long time and done in silos — challenges in maintaining up-to-date skills and knowledge driven by rapid changes in science and technology.
5. Policy, regulatory practices, funding and investment models heavily weighted toward maintaining the status quo with insufficient sustainable incentives to stimulate innovations.
6. Integration difficulties are reinforcing fragmented health services.

Trade-off mindset

Many First world countries face demand pressure on health services from sicker and more complex patients driven by increasing and aging population, increasing and changing burden of diseases and significant changes in social determinants. At the same time aging and increasingly frustrated workforce, are working with service models, facilities and technologies that struggles to respond to demand pressures.

The result is growing gaps in outcomes, inequities and fiscal deficits. A commonly held view is that better outcomes and reducing inequities require additional funding for more services. Growing fiscal deficits in many First world countries like the UK and New Zealand reinforce the case for significant increases in funding.

However, even with increased funding, advancing all three objectives remains elusive especially when balancing the book objective is often seen as getting in the way of the other two objectives. The need for trade-off has taken hold amongst many current decision-makers and leaders. It is deemed impossible to deliver on all three objectives as increases in funding have not and unlikely in the future to keep up with changes in demand pressures.

Any future proof health system requires all three objectives to be advance concurrently as part of narrowing the chasm. Is this possible when First world health systems are now either operating in the narrowing of the gap before the tipping point (about to fail) or the widening of the gap beyond the tipping point (starting to fail)?

What many present-day decision makers fail to understand is "trade-offs" do not help to narrow or eliminate the widening chasm. At best it provides the illusion that we are doing something. Compromising on any of the three objectives will mean that any gains made will be unsustainable in the long run.

Pulling off this trifecta seems far away when one reads the commentaries of decision makers and leaders responsible for the current health system.
As many First world health systems come under pressure it is not a surprise that governments are under pressure from health professionals, administrators/managers, unions, academics, NGOs, employers and providers to increase funding with each Budget round. Commentators and advocates often cite measures such as % of the health budget to GDP, health funding per person and % of the health budget to the overall government budget to support the case for more government funding. Yes, more resources are essential and helps but insufficient to cross this chasm.

It is first and foremost a leadership challenge. We need leaders and decision makers that can meet the exponential effects of today's demand challenges and bring disruptive rather than linear changes to health services delivery that can close these gaps and cross the ever-widening chasm. Leaders we need to do this starts with an uncompromising positive mindset that the three objectives is non-negotiable and is singularly focused on what needs to be done to make it a reality.

What is the way forward?

Leading, managing and changing responses in an environment of exponential change requires more than just more funding, better strategy, tools, and resources. It needs leaders that can create a team-based culture and environment that is comfortable with constant change, prepared to take a safe to fail (early, fast and inexpensive) portfolio approach to innovation and courageous to make swift deliberate decisions (stop, accelerate or change) on current core activities.

Crossing the chasm to deliver on all three objectives requires the following 7 pieces of the jigsaw:

1. Change in mindset - from deficit to abundance, from risk to opportunities, from failure to learnings, from "me" to "us" from "blaming others to taking responsibility" and from "yes but" to "yes and."
2. System approach to a dual transformation change programme.
3. Integrated change framework to execute the change.
4. Different capability, capacity, skills, and knowledge for each part of the dual transformation.
5. Open, learning, team-based and courageous culture.
6. Keeping pace with changes in external environment.
7. Making changes internally to be ahead of external environment changes.

Final remarks

The three objectives of "better outcomes, reducing inequities and balancing the books" is the high water mark for any health system. Today's ever-growing and deepening chasm between the exponential forces that drive demand and the linear pace of responses has given rise to a mindset that all three cannot be achieved. Trade-offs between them have to be made. This is flawed thinking and is an admission that the pressure has got the better of us. This flawed position is also contributing, reinforcing and deepening the chasm.

The alternative and only viable view, is to not just cross the chasm but always to be ahead of the demand curve so that ALL three objectives are a reality. The transition phase may see uneven progress, but the trend of improvements for all three objectives remains positive. Keeping the balance and ensuring that no one objective is lagging too far behind is complex and is first and foremost a leadership challenge.

Many government committees, boardroom, and senior executives agenda give an insight of where they are on this leadership challenge. There are glimpses of progress but there remains a lot of ground to be covered. When you read this article, where are you and your organization in this leadership challenge? Reflect on where you and your organisation are currently position on the exponential/linear graph and against the 7 pieces of the jigsaw puzzle. History are made and futures shaped by those who embrace and execute all 7 pieces of the jigsaw!

Chapter XIII

-

Better Care For Seniors

Key To Solving The Sustainability Of Health Systems

by Chai CHUAH

Executive summary

This article explores why finding new and better ways to support and care for seniors holds the key to solving First world countries health and social care services sustainability dilemma.

Most First world countries are racing against time to find credible and sustainable solution for their struggling health and social care system. Countries like France, UK, Germany, Japan, USA, Canada, Australia and New Zealand regardless of how well there are funded faces this growing tipping point challenge.

One of the common themes for First world countries health and social care system is the increasing demand pressure from ***aging, aged or super aged*** population. For many of these countries it translates into constant and unrelenting pressure to increase funding and resources for more services. The current higher percentage of health and social care spending on seniors compared to average is a major contributor to the current service and fiscal pressure in many First world countries. This will increase exponentially to an unsustainable level in the next 5, 10 to 30 years if nothing changes.

Talk to any experienced healthcare clinicians or other frontline carers and they will tell you that they are caring for more and older seniors. Many are also sicker and require more support to remain independent. It is therefore not surprising that this population group currently consume proportionately significant higher level of expenditure compared to other population groups.

Despite the dedication and commitment of many frontline staff and carers there is an increasing and loud disquiet about access, choice and quality of care for seniors. Mainstream media both print and digital runs disturbing and sometimes graphic stories of poor care either in nursing homes, supported living, primary care and in hospitals. One of the common theme from these stories is that it is the family members (many are seniors themselves) that are raising concerns on the poor care for their parent generation. This growing dissatisfaction and frustration of this "new seniors" should not be underestimated as a key catalyst for significant change.

Today's consumer networks for baby boomers' new seniors have similarities with traditional advocacy groups. The main difference is how they are using smart technology to express and share their views and resources with speed and reach a wider audience.

Any re-designing and implementation of new services need the active partnership and participation of seniors and be anchored on "values" principles fundamental to seniors. Health and social care institutions and decision makers will need to learn from other sectors that has successfully activated strong consumer networks. Such activation creates ownership and value of solutions from consumers.

There is no doubt that smart consumer focus technology will feature strongly in new services. These technologies are unlikely to totally replace human carers but rather it will augment and support future models of care. Apart from technology other changes needed to support future models of care includes changes to policies, regulation, funding, use of Big data and advance data analytics, augmented and new workforce and new business models.

 This article explores four significant themes in many First world countries:

1. The silver tsunami numbers
2. Increasing disquiet amongst seniors and their families – a catalyst for change
3. Unsustainability of current health and social care system to care for seniors.
4. Better ways of caring and supporting our seniors.

The silver tsunami numbers

The silver tsunami relates to the significant number of baby boomers reaching retirement age. When it comes to statistics and numbers on the silver tsunami there are three key numbers to focus on.

- The number and percentage of over 65s to total population.
- The **velocity** of aging (how fast the percentage is increasing).
- The number and percentage of over 80s to total population

The first number is the most common cited number. However it is equally important to look at the second and third number to get a comprehensive insight into the challenges ahead.

The second number is important because it provides the window available to respond to the change.

The third number is important because many of these over 80s seniors currently live most of their remaining years in poor health. This then drives exponential increases in health and social care services for seniors well past their 80th birthday.

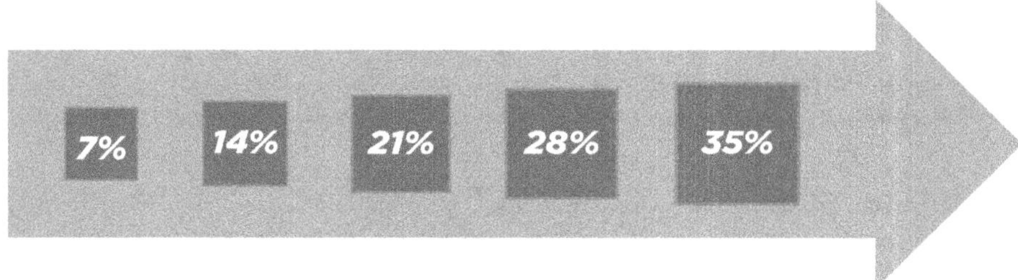

Graphic 3 - Over 65s - aging, aged, super aged, ultra-super aged societies and beyond!

Common working definition for **aging society** is where the population of over 65s make up more than **7%** of total population. Likewise an **aged society** is over **14%, super aged society** is over **21%** and an **ultra-super aged society** is over **28%**. There is no working definition yet when the percentage gets beyond **35%** (perhaps **mega-ultra-super aged**), yet a number of First world countries (Korea, Greece, Portugal, Spain and Japan) are forecast to 2050 to exceed this threshold.

Currently many First world countries are an aging and aged society. There are a few who are already a super-aged society. Traditionally two factors are driving this trend, a reducing birth rate and increasing life span. However, a third factor, migration is becoming a strong driver in recent years for some First world countries.

Based on an OECD 2017 report (here after referred to as the OECD report) in 2015 there were 4 countries that are "super-aged" societies with no countries in the "ultra-super-aged" or "mega-ultra-super-aged" categories. By 2050, there will be 22 "super-aged countries", "10 ultra-super-aged countries" and "5 mega-ultra-super-aged countries".

All things being equal, as countries move along the aging, aged, super-aged, ultra-super-aged and mega-ultra-super-aged continuum, the proportion of health and social care expenditure for their seniors will increase exponentially. This trajectory could get to a staggering unsustainable level and it will be hard to imagine what the health and social spending will look like for these countries.

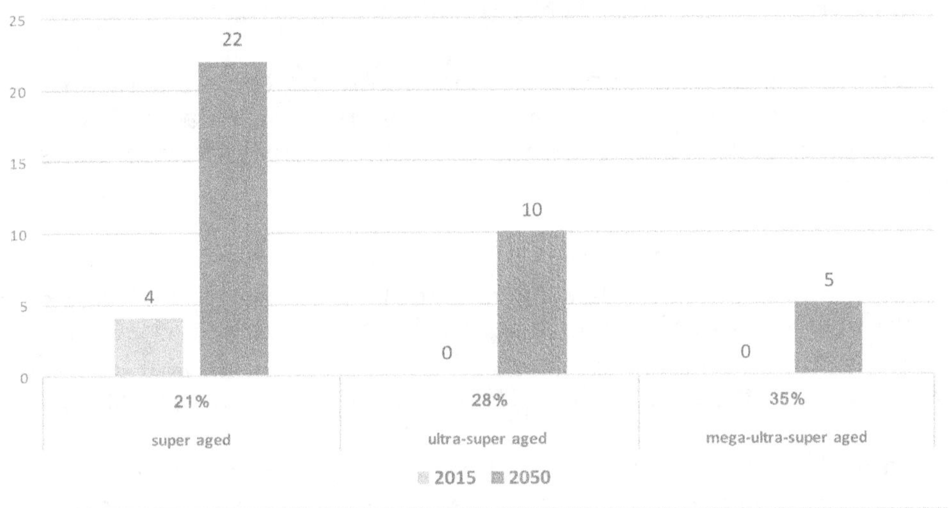

Graphic 4 - Super-aged, ultra-super-aged, mega-ultra-super-aged countries by 2015 and 2050.

Velocity of the aging

For some countries this number is critical. Currently they maybe have a relatively lower number for the population over 65s, it is how fast their population is aging that is of grave concern. Two clear examples Korea and China. Their over 65s will reach 35.8% and 26.3% in 2050 compared to 12.3% and 9.6% in 2015 respectively. This gives them a much smaller window to get prepared for that future. It will be beneficial to keep an eye on the responses from both these countries in the foreseeable future to meet their silver tsunami challenge.

Seniors 80 years and older - living longer but more years in poor health

Advances in medicine and public health have successfully prevented and cured major illness and diseases that contributed to increasing life expectancy in many countries.

According to an OECD report in 2015 there are no countries where 80 years and older exceeds 10% of its population. By 2050 however, 15 countries cross the 10% threshold, 13 in Europe, 2 in Asia (Japan and Korea) and 1 in North America (Canada).

While the average life expectancy is increasing this does not mean that they are living these longer years in good health. Growing number of seniors living longer are living many of these years in **poor health**.

An OECD report shows for 25 European countries at age 65 the average life expectancy is approximately 19 years and average healthy life expectancy is approximately 9 years. That means there is approximately **10 years** of these European seniors **living with poor health** or disabilities that limit an active and healthy life.

Longer life expectancy currently can bring with it increasing and often multiple chronic conditions as seniors get older. In addition, older seniors can often have increasing sight, hearing, strengthen, , continence, balance and mobility limitations that can rapidly lead to loss of independence. Therefore the need for more health and social care support increases significantly as seniors get older.

Unfortunately current health and social care systems are not able to cope with these demands. This growing chasm between growing and changing expectations of seniors (and their families) and the rate of change in health and social care services has two glaring consequences:

1. Increasing disquiet from seniors & their families
2. Unsustainable mounting pressure on both health and social care to provide services for seniors

Increasing disquiet from seniors & their families – a catalyst for change

In First world countries while many seniors receives great care and are grateful for the support they receive from dedicated and caring health professionals and carers it is not difficult to find on media both print and digital disturbing and sometimes graphic stories of how health and social care systems are failing our seniors.

Stories of neglect, abuse, medication errors, falls, malnutrition, neglect and financial affordability for seniors in care are familiar themes. Such stories for example in the aged care sector in Australia have prompted the Australian Prime Minister to launch a royal commission of inquiry recently. Even in countries that are "well-funded" for example both Germany and Japan health system are under pressure from workforce shortage.

Family members (many are baby boomers) of seniors in care are raising concerns and expressing lack of confidence in the health and social care system caring for their parent generation. This growing dissatisfaction and frustration of the baby boomer generation of "new seniors" will become a key catalyst for significant change.
What's behind the increasing disquiet from seniors and their seniors? The current health and social care system have focus largely on the functional well-being and needs of seniors. However, increasingly other fundamental unmet expectations are fuelling the seniors and their families disquiet and frustrations.

Beyond the physical and functional needs – what matters to seniors!

Some fundamental unmet expectations for seniors and their families includes, to remain connected, to contribute, be valued, independence, choice and control, belonging to a community, to be treated with respect and dignity.

These fundamental expectations become more important as seniors come to terms with diminishing mobility, hearing, sight, cognitive abilities and physical health. One of the more significant decisions often as a consequence of these diminishing capabilities is alternative living arrangements. Downsizing and shifting out of family homes are significant decisions for seniors and their families and can be difficult times for all. For seniors without children such time presents different challenges. Baby boomers as they go through the decision making process with their parents are thinking through for themselves how they might want to handle this transition differently when their time comes.

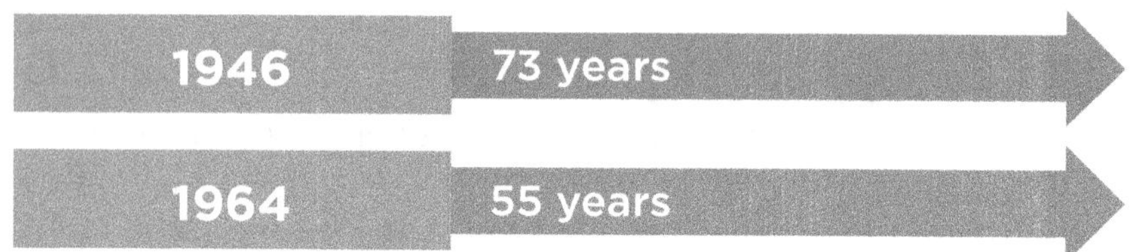

Graphic 5 - The mean age of baby boomers in 2019

Baby boomers – the new senior

Baby boomers are born in the two decades after the Second World War (1946 to 1964) and in 2018 the oldest and youngest baby boomers turned 72 and 54 respectively. Compared to their parent generation there are some important points to bear in mind about this generation:

1. More are mentally and physically active and on average at least half of baby boomers are still in active workforce. For example in the US, 2 out of 3 baby boomers are still in active workforce.

2. On average baby boomers have greater wealth and higher income per person. For example in Australia and UK they make up 25% and 30% of the population respectively but own over 50% of the total nation's wealth. In the US, boomers make up 24% of population and account for 47% of total income.

3. Many are open-minded and embrace new technology and social media.

4. Some baby boomers for different reasons are not part of or not up to-date with the digital society. Some baby boomers will rely largely on government retirement payments and services to support when they retire. In the US for example about 50% of baby boomers will fall into this category. They should not be forgotten or left behind.

It is not uncommon to hear baby boomers after a bruising experience in arranging care for their parents say "I am not going to allow this to happen to me. I have started to look at better options now rather leave it to others to decide for me".

Baby boomers are increasingly turning to modern technologies and the web to obtain information, share and express their views. Emails, Facebook and LinkedIn are most popular with this generation. A Forbes 2018 article reports that in Netherlands for example over 75% of baby boomers use Facebook, 89% of baby boomers have personal email accounts and of these 82% have at least one or more social media account.

The already exists numerous websites, blogs and online communities focusing on baby boomers for example SilverEco, Startsat60, Elder One Stop, Senior Planet and Silvernest. It is not beyond the realms of possibility that in the not too distant future ecommerce giants partnering with these organisations will make an entry into the health and social care services for seniors. After all they are already entering the health market in screening, diagnostics, primary care and some treatment therapies. With the right partners such networks and platforms have the potential to directly drive change in health and social care services.

Unsustainability of current health and social care system to care for seniors

Currently in most First world countries the health and social care expenditure per person for seniors is much higher than for the average person. In 2017 UK seniors make up 18.2% of the population and account for 66% of health expenditure. Likewise for Canada, in 2015 seniors make up 16.5% of the population and account for 46% of health expenditure. This pattern will be similar for most First world countries.

As these countries move up the aging, aged, super-aged, ultra-super-aged to mega-ultra-super-aged curve, it unrealistic to imagine that these countries can afford to carry on providing and funding health services in the same way. For politicians and policy makers there is more at stake beyond the fiscal risk.

The good news is the baby boomers new senior wants this sorted as well and can play a much more significant role in finding new and better solutions.

Pressure on health and social care services

Ask any frontline health staff working in First world healthcare system and they will tell you that the average age of patients continue to increase, generally sicker and with multiple chronic conditions.

Hospitals are now routinely caring for seniors in their 80's and well into their early 90's. Even in surgical wards the average age is also increasing as some seniors over 90 are receiving major joints procedures such as hips and knees replacements.

Rehabilitation services such as physiotherapy, occupational and speech therapies are also facing increasing demand from seniors recovering from surgery, stroke, heart attacks and falls.

Primary care like their hospital colleagues is also now caring for older seniors with multiple chronic conditions. Most of their senior patients are on multiple medications that need careful management especially when patients are being referred to or discharged from hospital care.

In nursing homes, aged residential care facilities as well as home support services for seniors, this increasing complexity of seniors needs has also not gone unnoticed. The higher level of disabilities and dependencies are requiring workforce with greater knowledge, skill and expertise.
Ambulance and patient transport services also face increased demand as seniors are unable to drive or arrange alternative transport to get to health facilities. Older seniors with increased disabilities are requiring additional and higher skill and knowledge from attending staff.

Increased cases of dementia amongst seniors require more social care and psychogeriatric support for them and their families.
Understandably many if not all of the above services continue to ask for more funding to be able to adequately resources more services to meet increased complexity and demand. Needless to say no jurisdiction to-date has adequately met these funding expectations.

Inquiries and reviews are the normal start points for many governments. There are two big issues with this traditional responses, one the recommendations are predictable largely focus on more funding, more staff, more facilities, tinker with organisational and structural change and maybe appoint some oversight commission or ombudsman. The second issue is while waiting for these reviews and subsequent recommendations to navigate its way through political priorities, public services policy and machinery of government processes, appropriation of funding, contracting providers with right capacity and capability to deliver new or expand existing services the chasm continues to grow. Better ways of caring and supporting our seniors cannot just be left alone to the usual incumbents and decision makers. It is not just the how and what needs to be done but who needs to be driving this.

Better ways of caring and supporting our seniors

New and better models of care for seniors are needed right across the care continuum from self-care to end of life care. There already exists interesting and innovative models that demonstrate direction of travel envisage in this article.

In self-care and home support, the recent explosion of self-monitoring wearables and use of sensors is gaining acceptance. Basic monitoring functions such as weight, diet, exercise, sleep and heart rate now comes as part of many smart mobile devices. The use of mobile devices for multi-media communication and connection is becoming a norm. The use of household, social and service robots (Paro, Pepper) for self-care and home support is emerging and wide spread adoption can be expected within the next 10 years.

In residential care, initiatives like De Hogeweyk dementia village in Netherlands, Aalborg Care Consortium development in Denmark, Beacon Hill village in USA and HOMESHARE in Australia are attracting new interests. On the back of these exemplars other innovative solutions are emerging including the University of Wollongong 700 hectares intergenerational connectivity project due to open in2022. Smart technology is and will continue to play a big part of future innovations and places like Shintomi Nursing Home in Japan showcase what is possible with their use of over 20 different types of social and service robots.

In primary care and hospital care, initiatives such as advance care directives and community based palliative care model needs greater tractions to avoid unnecessary medical treatment especially in the last year of life. The deployment of smart technology in primary care and hospitals to improve the care experience and provide seniors with more convenience, choice and control are right direction of travel. In the next 10 to 20 years advances in genetic screening and editing will offer new options that will be more personalised, less invasive and minimise unnecessary treatments.

It will also be interesting to keep an eye out in Asia especially in Japan, Korea and China as they come to grips with what it takes to care for their rapidly aging population. World Health Organisation predicts that by 2030 these three Asian countries will have health care workforce shortfall of 1.4 million. Japan with the highest percentage of senior population have been and is experiencing the realities of caring for a super-aged society. Confronting insights such as "kudokushi" or the phenomenon of elderly dying alone and remain undiscovered for long period of time has sparked significant initiatives to care for their seniors. One such initiative is the increase use of technologies including automation, sensors, wearables, exoskeletons and robotics as they forecast huge shortage of human workforce. A recent 2018 Nuffield report "What can England learn from the long-term care system in Japan?" provides useful insights of how Japan cares for their seniors.

Underlying "values" principles

Development and implementation of new services need to be underpin by "values" principles that are important to seniors. These include:

1. Dignity, respect, independence, security, cultural context, contribution, companionship, choice, control and sense of being part of a community.
2. Well-being is about the reasons one wishes to be alive. Early discussion on why and what seniors want to achieve rather than just focusing on functional needs.

3. Deliberate activation and partnership with seniors in any design process.

4. Dual purpose of improving services for those receiving them AND increasing access for those currently missing out especially for the most vulnerable seniors.

5. Improvement should result in strengthening and simplifying the wider system supporting seniors.

Managing change and transition – strengthen the "relevant" current and creating the "new"

Scaling existing and new innovative models is the fundamental issue in almost all health systems. A common assumption is that it is largely a question of funding. While funding is an issue, there are other more significant drivers that need to be addressed including changes to organisation and business models, policies and regulation. Finally and probably the most deciding factor in managing successful transition is the new talent, capabilities, capacities, skills and knowledge to manage the change and transition.

Careful transition will be needed to both improve current service models where it is still relevant and create new and better models. The best of the current models need to be retained and improved, while others will need to be discontinued.

Within current models courageous leadership is needed to execute what one Health Affairs article calls the 6 categories of waste (overtreatment, failures of care coordination, failures in execution of care processes, administrative complexity, pricing failures, and fraud and abuse). The same article estimates that wastage is at least 20% of total health expenditure. It is not uncommon to hear those currently in charge to say "there is no more efficiencies left, any further cuts will result in compromising patient safety and the real problem is that it is a lack of funding!" That is why these 6 categories of waste are unlikely to be realised by incumbents if that is their starting position.

Creating and implementing new services is the second part of this transition. This is about creating and developing new services not re-engineering or changing or modifying existing services.

Different talent, capabilities, capacities, skills and knowledge are needed compared to what is needed to manage or improve current services.

How incumbents make this transition will almost entirely be dependent on the quality of their organisation leaders, their awareness of seismic and rapid changes taking place around them and their ability to appropriately respond. Too often managing change also suffers from a lack of discipline in implementation and inappropriate knowledge and use (sometimes none at all) frameworks and tools. Without a sound understanding of the complexity of presenting challenges and the use of appropriate tools and frameworks, implementation takes too long, ineffective and fails to make any impact.

Useful frameworks

Some useful frameworks to provide a discipline approach to support development and implementation of new services include:

• Complex change requires a "discovery approach" to implementing portfolio of safe to fail initiatives. Complicated and simple change can benefit from good practice and best practice but are inappropriate for complex change.

• An integrated reform in four key domains for change to be sustainable:
>	1) New Service Model
>	2) New policies, regulatory and funding regimes
>	3) New organisation and business models
>	4) New enablers & resources (workforce, IT, facilities, devices, data)

• The 10%, 20%.30% and 40% of change:
>	1) 10% being the good idea
>	2) 20% is the passionate leadership
>	3) 30% is the organisation culture, talent, capacity, and capability
>	4) 40% is the operating environment and context at local to international levels

• Disruptive change to solve unmet need requires:

1) New partners. They must share not just the same ambition but also the same values. Some must come from outside the health sector

2) New networks. This is necessary to mitigate barriers from mainstream networks that will be difficult or costly to access.

3) New organisation and business models. They mean different things. Of particular interest will be the platform organisation models and the complementary platform business models

4) New talent, capabilities, capacities, skills and knowledge for improving current services as well as creating new services.

5) Focus on the edge and margin. Look for where the edges are. It is where there is currently significant unmet need. At the edge, mainstream and incumbents are paying least attention.

6) New services design to reach those consumers currently missing out need to be affordable and initially do not need all the bells and whistles.

New entrants collaborating with like-minded health care sector players

A big part of the new and better models of care for seniors is to take a broader system view of well-being. This includes making changes to, connecting with the broader determinants of well-being including housing, utilities, transport, diet and social interactions.

Many of these services are already being provided by ecommerce organisations. It should not be a surprise that in the near future these non-health sector players collaborating with like-minded health care sector partners are likely to drive many of these disruptive changes in the health care sector. Successful ecommerce organisations are good at engaging and improving consumers' experience, use of modern technologies and have an appetite to innovate and enter new sectors including the healthcare market. The entry of Amazon, Berkshire and JP Morgan into the US healthcare market and their appointment of Dr Atul Gawande as CEO is the most obvious example of such an approach.

Conclusion

Solving and finding better ways to care for seniors holds the key to a sustainable future for health and social services. The catalyst for this change is a growing disquiet and frustration of seniors and their families coupled with the entrance of new players partnering with liked minded incumbents that understand how to harness consumer power. The development of new and better models of care and associated business models will happen and will be disruptive. The challenge of managing the transition of this disruptive change is to make sure in maximising the benefits and minimising the cost, the gains are inclusive, equitable and sustainable.

Change has to take place right across the continuum from self-care to palliative care. Retaining, improving and eliminating the wastage from the best of current services are necessary but not sufficient. New and better service models supported by appropriate business models need and will emerge. This is unlikely to happen if left to the current decision makers and vested interest running the system. That is why seniors especially the baby boomers cannot sit back but have to drive this change as consumers.

Section-III:
Realities will drive future

Chapter XIV

-

Hospital Of The Future

by Dr. H. Omer TONTUS

"Hospitals should transition from being "the last link in a chain" of health service providers to being actively engaged with their communities and with providers of primary care. Altering the traditional model starts with discarding an emphasis on "filling the beds" in favor of a new role of hospitals as part of collaborative networks."

(C. Etienne, Chicago 2015)

Just before start "imagine the future of the possible", and try to answer the following question;
How could digitally integrated technological tools help patients in the course of the care process from admission to discharge, and from post-discharge care services to follow-up?

Within a decade, new technologies, digital transformation and IoMT "can" and "will" change every aspect of global healthcare service delivery.

In the healthcare sector, the cost of service or care continue to rise, and many healthcare providers are seeking long-term solutions to minimize inpatient services and their cost. In this chapter, we will try to find answers to the following question; "how new technologies and healthcare service will merge to penetrate the future of hospital design and the patient experience across the globe?".

Themes for the hospital of the future

Probably, in future hospitals, healthcare services delivery will be entirely different than today's hospital. Advancing technologies, alongside with demographic and socio-economic changes, are expected to modify healthcare institutions globally. In general, as the level of health literacy in society increases, individuals take more responsibility for their health. This enables some health services to be offered at home. Therefore, an increasing number of inpatient healthcare services are being forced into home and outpatient clinics. However, plenty of complicated and critical patients will persist to demand inpatient services.

In many countries, due to obsolete and aged hospital infrastructure and more bed demand, governments are taking account integrating digital technologies into conventional hospital services to optimize inpatient and outpatient settings and to create a healthcare system without barrier.

To understand what future of health care delivery will look like, I personally analyzed literature written by healthcare leaders, physicians, public policy leaders, WHO experts, digital technologists, and futurists. Articles were explaining the design of digital hospitals globally next two decades with specific cases.

As can be understood from the literature reviews, we can classify the main headings as follows:

1. Innovations in healthcare service delivery:

Including "healthcare data centers" to enable data mining for better decision making, continuous clinical monitoring, target cell focused marked drugs, 3D tissue printing, portable diagnostic devices, pre-hospital clinical decision-making processes will help and stimulate future acute-care hospitals.

Future hospitals will be monitored digitally by a central control unit (CCU). For example, in online shopping via Amazon, the product is taken from the shelf in the warehouse, placed on the conveyor belt, reaching to the packaging unit, packing it, adhering the correct address label and directing it to the right cargo unit is already done with digital technologies. All these steps are controlled by a digitalized central unit. Same will happen to hospitals, such as directing the people in front of a concentrated department in hospitals, providing the equipment needed during an endoscopic procedure, directing the necessary support personnel, changing the appointment order which is deteriorated due to long-term operation. Performing these procedures very quickly will be provided by the digitalization of the system. For these procedures, CCUs need collecting processable data through new technologies to manage such and similar operations. Currently, a similar digital control unit is used by Cleveland Clinic. Today, in all hospitals, every procedure from patient records to laboratory results, from MRI imaging to invoicing, generates digital data. The use of digital technology systems that will process this data and support the decision process will be a necessity for future hospitals. These units will also serve as an early warning system against possible threats. For example, CCU will turn off the lights of a corridor without mobility, will turn off the air conditioner of the room if the windows open, and will inform the related department of a medical device failure.

Such technologies will make in-hospital processes instantaneous and proactively manageable. For example, regular follow-up of blood glucose levels and making insulin injections in the required dose can be performed by using wearable devices for follow-up of diabetic patients. Real-time data from these kinds of devices will be controlled by the dedicated CCU. Wearable devices will be possible to use in patients with cardiac arrhythmia, hypertension, motor dysfunction (fall risk), and data collected from these devices will be monitored instantaneously by AI. Thus, effective and timely service delivery will be provided to more patients without increasing work load. Big data analysis, integration of digital technology such as ML, AI, CCU "will allow caregivers to have a chance to intervene individuals without experiencing a potential health problem" and "will lead to a more effective management of hospitals".

2. Personalized healthcare:

A number of new technological advances, such as 3D tissue printing, robotic or micro-robotic applications, nanotechnology, genetic coding or cloning, can provide individual patient care and make the service more accessible. Think about, the heart rhythm monitoring devices (Holter monitor) which are used just last decade ago and which require a bag to carry, are now available as wearable such as a watch. As in this example, many devices are becoming smaller and more portable. This will turn into the form of a mobile mini-clinic that tracks all the health data from the individual to produce unique solutions. In this way, the treatments will probably become more targeted, and future health services will be instantly available and more sensitive, personalized. By these kinds of changes, the collected data will give clinicians the opportunity to apply the best treatment option quickly rather than "try and see" treatment options. Thus, the timely and unique treatment will be offered to the patient while increasing the efficiency of the staff and the process. In the following decade, personalization of the drugs in relevant with the genetic profile of the patient will be provided, and prostheses (such as hip or dental prosthesis) will be produced by 3D printing technology during the surgical procedure in accordance with the patient's specific anatomy.

The shrunk medical equipment size (as an example, consider the size of ECG devices 20 years ago and today's mobile-phone sized

ECG devices) and new highly sensitive sensors are developed to become more portable. In this way, more and more equipment can be transported to the patient's bedside, instead of mobilizing patients to different areas of the hospital for various procedures. Programmable wearable robotic devices for patients receiving regular medications at regular intervals may be used to administer medication. These kinds of changes will give opportunities for personalized healthcare.

3. Cloud-based EHR / EMR solutions:

The electronic health records or electronic medical records are likely to be the main element of decision support systems at the future hospital by processing data of different sources. Combined with AI, the use of EHR can create process efficiency and facilitate decision making to improve quality. The collected data can be better integrated into daily care and patients can play a role in determining their own data as well as their own health.

Real-time patient data can improve patient outcomes by guiding better care. Also, sharing standard data can be part of the delivery of in-hospital or out-of-hospital care in the future. EHR / EMR data may include genetic, demographic, social and behavioural information about patients, as well as financial, clinical, and administrative records. The data can be safely stored in the cloud-based so that it is accessible when needed. This allows easy access to data from multiple locations and devices at a lower cost, and also enables the consultant physicians to see the patient's information when transferring a patient to a referral hospital without file transfer during a referral process before patient reach.

With a large amount of data flow, many hospitals will need cognitive analyses for data sorting and they will detect the most essential personalised points and trends. These detections can be proactively presented to physicians, patients, and other related healthcare providers in an easy-to-understand format for their daily activities to be carried out without problems. By EHR, patients can own data related to themselves. They can add new health records to their own data, edit existing data and communicate proactively with their physicians. Importantly, the data will not be open to unauthorized personnel even for research purposes.

4. Artificial Intelligence technologies for better patient satisfaction in hospital of future:

Artificial intelligence (AI) technologies can facilitate on-demand reciprocal actions and smooth processes to make better patient satisfaction.

Future hospitals will be better in informing and educating patients, alleviating anxiety, and enabling them to actively participate in care before, during and after hospitalization.

Since the early 2000s, individuals around the world are familiar to get instant and quick information about news, weather forecasts, concerts, or holiday packages. Many people want to find answers to their health-related questions at the same speed. Every day, an increasing number of individuals are being online to learn about healthy lifestyles, diseases and treatment options.

In the near future, digital technologies will evolve people's experience by providing real-time access to medical information. Hospitals will need an AI-assisted bedside virtual care assistant which can categorize and respond to patients' questions. This AI based virtual assistants can answer common basic questions about the patient's diagnosis, treatment times, treatment options and daily medication programs. Additionally, this virtual assistant can serve as a data store for the patient's medical background, laboratory results, consultation dates and notes, appointments, and even contribution of other patients with identical symptoms. Such accessible in-hospital AI-assisted programs still in use in some of the institutions are providing great support to patients and their families. The AI virtual assistant can partially produce solutions to the lack of professional human resources, which is considered to be the most important problem of the health system in the future. The simple questions of patients and their relatives may be intense enough to prevent health workers from producing health care. The fact that every hospitalized patient takes the time of the health worker for every question he/she wants to ask questions constitutes an obstacle to the sustainability of the service. AI-assisted technologies provide answers that can help patients relax, also if required it canalizes the question to the right person to find best answers. Thus, unnecessary waste of time for health professionals is prevented by AI.

Hospitals are often stumbled in admissions and discharge procedures, especially in operational performance and patient experience. Patients frequently complain about filling the documents which are requesting similar entry in every admission or discharge processes. While hospital procedures are digitalized, personnel can use AI technologies to help learn and improve processes and help patients use it.

I can easily say that in the near future there will be no patient registration process. By AI technologies, when a doctor offers hospitalization, or when a doctor approves the hospitalization via software, all the patient admission procedures are carried out and a personalized hospitalization welcome information package is shared with the patient. Any kind of required clinical, financial and demographic information of the patient can be filled with the pre-existing records on the system. These records can be cloud-based and easily accessible by process stakeholders according to their authorization level. The AI included in the process can help physicians, healthcare personnel and patients for selecting the room type, storing the necessary drugs, identifying the diagnostic options and providing non-medical support based on the patient's socio-demographic profile.

AI processes can be connected with the discharge workflow. Typically, today's practice, nurses or caregivers offer specific information to patients based on their clinical condition, medical background, behaviour and attitude. Some patients need more time than others for understanding and confirming the information made to them. Nurses often do not have enough time for patients' questions, as they often have to work on tasks with different priorities. When all information is collected in one place (cloud based), AI algorithms can be integrated into the virtual assistant to create customized discharge instructions that can be given to the patient during discharge for the recovery period. Patients can interact with AI-virtual assistant and ask questions, and if they need professional medical instructions, they can talk to nurses or other health personnel as long as they need to.

As stated, AI technologies simplify every procedure such as patients' hospitalization, discharge, diagnosis, referral and billing.

5. Enhanced recruiting, scheduling, learning and talent development with Intelligent personnel recruitment

Recruitment and scheduling can provide efficiency through the use of AI-analytics. Staff development departments of hospitals may focus on continuous learning through virtual simulations and web-enabled distance education.

Nurse and personnel turnover cycle is a challenge in hospitals and in countries, too. Fast staff turnover-time leads to quality health service delivery problems. Staffs are the biggest cost element of most hospitals, and the necessity to staff change in a short time creates a secondary cost due to the need for training. Digitalization and AI technologies may help solve this mentioned problem in the future.

Increasingly, the staff recruitment departments of hospitals are using cognitive analytics (CA) and robotic process automation (RPA) to help automate the selection process. Cloud-based AI solutions may help profiling and filter applicants easily and quickly so managers can choose the best applicants. AI-analytical technologies can automatically compare candidates' experience or academic level depending on the sector's realities and institutional structure. As a consequence of these processes, it plays an important role in deciding the candidate's salary, social rights and benefits.

Scheduling shifts are becoming more complicated, as the workforce moves toward a new era which workers with short-term contracts are more common than classic full-time workers. Also, with a continuing focus on better patient outcomes and improved patients' satisfaction worldwide, hospital executives will likely need to use AI-analytics for staff recruitment. The most appropriate staff placement can only be done according to well-analyzed patient expectations, audit and satisfaction data. AI technologies are required for this. AI also can help staffing optimization with reduced unplanned overtime and can help organize staff contracting.

While AI technologies with IoT and cognitive analytics can track performance management for staff, IoT and RFID instruments can track personnel activities such as time of arrival and leave, number of patients they see, and the time spent for patients' care. Managers can then evaluate the data and determine where efficiency can be increased by the help of AI. While some personnel believe that these applications and instruments are intruded on their work, a barrier these can be overcome if the trust is established between managers and staff.

6. Virtual learning and development

Virtual training is becoming more popular day by day. While virtual training is being more common among students and experienced clinicians, personal medical practice training can never be eliminated. Virtual training helps surgeons develop skills and identify the techniques they will use before performing surgery. Virtual training also provides training to increase the level of expertise to a wider audience at the lowest cost without geographical boundaries.

Virtual training can be monitored by means of apps or other software and may foster healthcare professionals to keep up with their training needs. In addition, requirements can be linked to performance criteria based on objective criteria. According to the data obtained from the assessment methods, clinicians can be given courses in topics where they need supplementary training instead of the subjects they want to learn more. Many medical centers already use VR programs to train surgeons.

7. Robotic technologies and automation for healthcare and collateral services

The development of robotics and automation to trim inefficient processes can be resulted by reducing costs and improving revenue.

Within a typical hospital setting, laboratory samples, linens, supplies, medications, and other goods travel hundreds of kilometers in a week. That means hospitals also work as mini-logistics companies inside of their walls and they continuously move large volumes of material among units. While this logistics function has a cost, it is also one of the core facilities of hospitals to provide patient care. Nurses typically spend less than two hours of a 12-

hour shift on direct patient care (Rhonda Collins, 2007). According to a published study, nurses spend approximately 2-hour in 12-hour shift periods for direct patient care. During the remaining 10 hours of 12-hours shift, nurses are doing administrative work such as preparing medicines and finding supplies, coordinating laboratory needs and even dispense patient's meal.

The use of robots for automatizing of the hospital ancillary services and back-office works can provide significant cost and time efficiency and enhance reliability. With a simple command, nurses and other health personnel can invoke robotics technology for specific tasks. For example, robots can carry blood samples, collect laboratory or imaging results, and plan laundry and food delivery. Robotic processes can also be used for accounting and finance functions such as timing and claims processing.

8. Blockchain and contracting through new technologies:

Some hospitals have invested heavily in data and operations management systems for the electronic health record apps or software, supply chains, and revenue cycle over the past few years. Still, interoperability, cyber security, and inefficient processing persist to challenge the effectiveness of operation management of many hospitals.

In the UK, according to a survey conducted by the NHS revealed that more than half of respondents who work on acute care hospital encountered patient record access issues.16 In the USA, more than 75% of hospital directors stated that they utilize manual processes for their supply chains management, which can lead to excessive cost and data accuracy matters.17

Blockchain technologies have the potential to transform much of these procedures. Blockchain is a distributed, unchangeable entry of digital transactions that is shared amongst stakeholders. Blockchain's strength lies in its data integrity.

Some examples of how Blockchain can improve hospital management are listed below:

• Data interoperability: Blockchain can help "health information exchanges" with reducing fears of security.

• Supply chain management: Goods management of the hospital includes planning, purchasing, and tracking items stock (from medical supplies to drugs)

• Revenue cycle management: Applying blockchain to claims, adjudication and payment process systems can eliminate the need for intermediaries between the healthcare providers, doctors, insurance companies, and patients. It also helps to decrease managerial expenses.

Health Information Exchange (HIE) is a process of sharing patients' HER or EMR among healthcare providers and patients.

9. Healing and well-being designs of future hospitals

In spite of the patient-oriented designs, which have recently developed positively, most of the hospitals are stressful and boring. Hospital design can improve patient satisfaction and enhancement of personnel productivity. Hospitals will likely have special designs for patients' and personnel's well-being. Hospital managers increasingly accept that the design of the institution has a positive effect on physical and mental health and contribute to a faster recovery period with increased patients' satisfaction.

A hospital of the future design will incorporate the following features:

• Customized patient rooms: Peoples are changing their smartphone wallpaper often because they are bored to see the same picture every day. Same things happen to a patient after a week stay in a hospital room. The hospital environment can impact on the overall patient satisfaction with its design, negatively or positively. Instead, imagine a hospital room contains multiple LCD screens which are showing photos of the patient's family members, or pictures of the patient's best moments. In addition, a patient can organize a music list with own choice and make video calls with friends via web access provided by the hospital. Sensors can be integrated into bathrooms for monitoring abnormal activities such as fall. Probably, customized hospital rooms will be a standard concept in the hospital of the future.

• Smart and pleasant common areas: Future hospital will include attractive lounges, daily activity rooms, library and natural places (indoor green natural life imitations), healing horticultural environments. These can help reduce patient anxiety and promotes healing period.

• Management for better lighting and less noise: Easily scalable bright ambient lighting can bring significant change in patient-centred care. Appropriate lightings increase patient's satisfaction and experience and, especially in terms of mood and pain perception. There is growing literature that links between hospital noise (mostly caused by primarily staff conversation, alarms, and medical devices) and sleep interruption, increased BP, tachycardia. Hospitals in the future will offer noiseless acoustic engineering to eliminate ambient noise.

• Focus on safety: Hospitals are responsible for everyone's safety, as well as overcoming a great human mobility every day. Hospital staff need to be prepared for anything from vandalism to aggravated behaviour of patients and relatives. Hospitals now are using digital technologies to supplement physical security. There is an intention for systematic RFID tracking with tags for patients, personnel and equipment. Furthermore, AI connected security cameras are monitoring facial recognition and empathic expression detection for preemptive activity.

10. Increased operational efficiencies by multilateral technologies:

Digital technology driven operational efficiencies such as AI based supply chains, inventory management, procurement management, HR management, automation and robotics can promote management and back-office performance.

11. Healthy life style and well-being designs:

The wellbeing of patients and personnel will presumably be the central idea of future hospitals' design. With the increase of health literacy and digital technology literacy, individuals will choose healthy living culture habit and will participate in activities in this direction. In the hospital designs of the future, this habitual transformation will be the main concept of architectural design. The preservation of health and attitudes of healthy life focused hospital construction will dominate future instead of disease and treatment-oriented structuring.

Many of the changes mentioned above are still experienced. Hospital managers should plan how to integrate technology into newly built institutions and adapt them to older ones.

Technological infrastructure will form the background of future healthcare from hospital building to staff management. However, paying attention to certain complex cases and procedures will require practical human expertise.

In addition to that, since digital technologies are likely to play an important role in the future, as health services and diseases are absolutely unique to the individual, the caregiver factor especially for complex cases and procedures will be permanent in all healthcare sectors. For the upcoming two decades, probably, most of the procedures may still require hands-on healthcare professional expertise.

Conclusion:

As the healthcare system shifts toward paying for patient outcomes and satisfaction, hospitals will focus on reducing cost, improving quality, and boosting patients' experience.

The use of green space and more windows will open future hospitals to the outside, rather than closing them off like the institutionalized four-walled boxes of the past. Inside the hospitals, privatised patient rooms will have wide windows, comfortable furniture, and built-in bedside tablets for patient communication. As hospitals' "customers" shift from insurer to patients, more medical buildings will be designed to enhance the satisfaction of patients and their relatives.

Hospitals' online patient portals will allow patients to check in before patients show up for their procedure or hospital stay. And they will see their medical records and test results, wherever they are.

Patients will also be able to consult with a doctor or nurse by video or online chat before the drive to the emergency department or urgent care centre, if they need guidance. AI technologies and apps will grow rapidly for guiding the patient to the best parking spot and to the desired destination inside the hospital.

Hospitals spend a lot of money to take care of a patient admitted to the hospital, with the help of digitalisation hospitals will not need to keep patients long term.

Telehealth will allow hospitals to discharge patients earlier and monitor patients after discharge. While at home, patients will be monitored regularly with the help of a nurse or doctor via advanced communication technologies. If their health data changes or an in-person visit is needed, CCU will direct a mobile health team to visit the patients. Telehealth remote monitoring will keep an eye on patients' vital functions from the moment they hospitalized. If there's a problem caregivers can be directed immediately by CCU.

Technology will also help doctors' diagnose, free staff from administrative burdens, and manage operating costs more tightly. Big data analysis and artificial intelligence will shine in these areas. Also, hospitals will be categorized, one type of hospital will treat sicker or more acute care patients. These will probably be located at medical centres of universities or at well-established hospitals in an urban area. The other type is suburban and community hospitals. They will focus on preventive medicine, providing primary care services, taking care of patients with chronic illnesses, and performing common procedures.

In the future hospitals will specialize more, especially within large health systems where they can save money. Instead of every hospital in a health system having oncology, maybe there will be two or three hospitals that specialized in this field, and they will be geographically dispersed across the country. Hospitals will no longer try to provide all services but will be known for a few specialties. Above all, we know that the changes in the construction sector do not catch up with the speed of technologies developed to provide better health care. Therefore, when the construction of a hospital designed with a futuristic perspective is completed, many of its features will be outdated. Therefore, hospitals of the future will always be on the agenda.

References

1. Angela Dawson, Helen Stasa, Michael Roche, Caroline Homer and Christine Duffield, "Nursing churn and turnover in Australian hospitals: nurses perceptions and suggestions for supportive strategies," BMC Nursing 13:11 (2014) Doi: 10.1186/1472-6955-13-11

2. David Maguire; "Interoperability and the NHS: are they incompatible?" via The Kings Fund, August 08, 2016. https://www.kingsfund.org.uk/blog/2016/08/interoperability-and-nhs accessed January 23, 2019.

3. Deloitte: The hospital of the future; How digital technologies can change hospitals globally, https://www2.deloitte.com/global/en/pages/life-sciences-and-healthcare/articles/global-digital-hospital-of-the-future.html

4. Denise Choiniere, "The effects of hospital noise" Nursing Administration Quarterly 34, no. 4(2010): pp. 327—333. DOI: 10.1097/NAQ.0b013e3181f563db

5. Edwin Lopez, Jennifer McKecitt; "Survey: Hospital supply chain practices are outdated," Supply Chain Dive, February 21, 2017. https://www.supplychaindive.com/news/hospital-supply-chain-survey-cardinal-inventory/436505/ accessed May 19, 2019.

6. Rhonda Collins; "Bringing Nurses Back to the Bedside," For the Record, Vol. 27 No.9 P.10. https://www.fortherecordmag.com/archives/0915p10.shtml accessed January 23, 2019.

7. Roxanne Nelson "Personalized Medicine Delivers Better Outcomes: More Proof," via Medscape May 19, 2016, http://www.medscape.com/viewarticle/863499, accessed January 22, 2019.

8. Timothy Hsu, Erica Ryherd, Kerstin Persson Waye and Jeremy Ackerman, "Noise Pollution in Hospitals: Impact on Patients," The Journal of Clinical Outcomes Management 19, no. 7 (2012): pp. 301-309. https://pdfs.semanticscholar.org/27db/5536c0a580983f3efd1b30374f64cacacd65.pdf?_ga=2.47212900.2106118448.1559974100-370942572.1559974100 accessed January 22, 2019.

9. What Will Your Hospital Look Like in 5 Years? https://www.healthline.com/health-news/future-of-hospitals-in-five-years accessed March 9, 2019.

Chapter XV

-

Guiding Principles For The Designing Of The Digital Hospital Of Future

by Dr. H. Omer TONTUS

The digitalized hospital is a concept contributing to improving staff productivity, assisting hospital management, developing the operational quality, increasing patient satisfaction and providing patient safety by combining most advanced technologies such as wearable medical equipment, smart data management systems, facility control and automatic conveyor systems. It integrates location-based services, sensors, monitors and digital communication tools into healthcare service processes.

Building a digital hospital of the future requires changing investment models in individuals, public, technology, processes and buildings. Most of these changing will likely be evident and fast. In the short-term, investors might not see swift returns on these new models of investment. However, in the long-term, digitalization technologies can better healthcare services which resulted in higher patients' satisfaction, improve operational efficiency which resulted in higher better staff experience. Therefore, investors may see returns on investments as a result of increased care quality and better operational efficiency.

Listed core elements of digital strategy can help to push hospital into the future:

1. Creating a culture of digital transformation: It is essential that managers or investors understand the significance of the digital future and provides approval for the implementation of transformation at all institutional levels.

2. Considering technologies that communicate with each other: Digitalization is an absolute complicated process. Linking dissimilar apps, tools, and technologies all connected to each other and being confident they communicate with each other is crucial for an accomplished digital implementation.

3. Making a changeable long-term project plan: Because digital technologies are constantly progressing, flexibility and scalability can be critical in the course of implementation. The planning team for digitalization must be aware that the project scope includes "addition, extension, modification, or replacing technologies" at minimum costs.

4. Focusing on data for digitalization: Data can be measured, analyzed, directed to new developments, and can provide flexibility to change, so digitalization must be managed by data sources base. Data collection and processing are crucial for both the transformation period and the future.

5. Discovering and supporting talents: Adding digital technologies to future hospitals will require staff to use them. Existing employees need to be familiarized with digitalization in the process of change.

6. Ensuring cybersecurity: Any type of innovations brings new threats. The threat of possible cyber-attacks is an important issue that should not be ignored by managers of future hospitals. Cybersecurity should be comprehended as the other crucial half of digitalization and must be managed, properly by change supervisors or leaders.

Suggested steps to take

Medical technology is booming at a rapid pace progressively both in diagnose methods and treatment options as well as hospital instruments, equipment and tools. The complexity of data management, administrative duties and logistics processes are also increasing sharply. Modern information technologies provide the key to answering these challenges. Digitalization has been committed to this task and gave a chance to the creation of comprehensive products. Successful digitalization offers rapid, effective processing of hospitals' and patients' data, reducing workload for doctors and other medical personnel and generate cost-effectiveness advantage.

In the upcoming ten years, many hospitals' managers in the USA and Europa have plans to renovate, restore or reconstruct their aged infrastructure. Similarly, enlarging healthcare demand in developing countries could motivate a significant number of hospital constructions projects. For example, spending on new hospital projects in India is anticipated to reach $200 billions by 2024, and China has projects for adding 89,000 new hospital beds by 2020. The very early examples of future hospital projects were launched in Turkey. The construction period for 21 hospital campus project containing approximately 30,815 beds was started in mid-2016 with almost $6 Billion-dollar investment budget. Until May 2019, nine of them started to provide healthcare service and remaining will start to operate before end of the 2021. When the construction of the projects is completed, half of the total hospital beds will be new in Turkey. These projects have been planned in the new concept of digital hospital construction, not renovation nor re-construction. All of these hospital projects are future-oriented hospitals with digitalization and AI infrastructure and are good examples for other countries.

It is not necessary to wait for such a building boom "like Turkey did" to integrate new digital technologies into hospital operations. Some of the digitalization technologies don't require new bricks or big redesigning/reconstructing projects; they can be implemented directly to improve operational efficiencies and better clinical outcomes for higher patients' satisfaction.

Digitalization technologies solutions for hospitals should take the following steps:

• Digitally delivered care: To diminish cost, increase quality, improve objectives and enhance outcomes, hospitals may use the digital technological instruments as a solution. Distant patient monitoring, telehealth, AI-technologies, EHR and wearables equipment can transform today's hospitals towards a future's hospitals. Healthcare systems with integrated digital technologies engage with patients, for improved quality and outcomes in a cost-effective manner.

• Digitally empowered patients' satisfaction: Hospitals may boost the patients' satisfaction by adopting digital technologies to aid patient access by applications, internet interface, individualized digital tools. In addition, digital instruments, such as IoT, IoMT, AR, and VR can help personalized inpatient services.

• Digitalized operations: Most of the back-office functions (such as staffing, PR works and HR management) can have the advantage of robots, innovative AI-analytics, sensors, and automation to manage cost effectiveness. These are also can be digitalized by cloud-based processes to make functions safer and faster.

• The long-term success of the organization with a digital strategy: Healthcare institutions which integrate digitalization into extensive organizational functions can enhance the potential in long-term success.

• Creating a digital revolution culture: It is vital that the executives understand the significance of the digital future and put in practice for all institutional levels.

• Communicating technologies: Digitalization is a complex process. Connecting different apps, devices, and technologies and making certain that they talk to each other is critical to a successful digitalization.

• Making investments manageable: It is undeniable that the transformation process has a cost. Some services can be hired to avoid high capital needs.

• Planning the long implementation period: Planning should be done knowing that the process of transformation needs a period of time. Some applications may even be updated with new versions in the process. For this reason, it is necessary to be open to changes, new add-ons and new technologies.

• Accepting data as a core element: Digital data is vital to future hospitals and should build a strong data infrastructure. Data collection, storage, security and mining titles should be structured on a sound basis. Hospitals should be creative for a potent data infrastructure.

• Maintaining cybersecurity: With the widespread of digital technologies, infringement can be a major risk to future hospitals' digital infrastructures. Cybersecurity is a "sine qui non" part of digitalization.

Suggestions for changes in design of the digital hospital of future

Nowadays, some hospitals are using the most advanced technologies that until recently were only seen in fiction. Using the latest technology, from Google Glass to 3D printing, hospitals can be named as "the hospital of the future" continues to offer treatment modalities to the patients, with some of the latest and best that medical technological options. But governments and investors may seek to participate in more Evidence-Based Design (EBD) research as a means of contributing to the hospital design and construction practices associated with improving the patients' experience. Researchers in the medical field can collaborate with design and construction researchers to find new ways in which digitalisation integrated designs can help improve patient outcomes. Similarly, design and construction researchers can work in partnership with medical researchers to determine how the latest design and digital technology can be put to use to improve healthcare.

In addition, design and digitalization research in healthcare will bridge the gap between the researchers making new discoveries and this will lead to the ultimate implementation of those findings in practice. Progress comes as a result of taking the ever-advancing knowledge and technology available to us and putting it to good use. Enhanced cooperation between AI technology experts, futurists and healthcare industry professionals across disciplines and specialties can accelerate the progress of healthcare facilities.

Conclusion
The digital hospital of the future: putting it all together

In the past, governments or investors have been considering the number of beds in hospital project planning. However, the number of beds is not a primary consideration for future hospital designing. Many health systems such as UnitedHealth Group, USA, Aetna, USA, or IHH Berhad, Malaysia are shifting their planning purpose with focusing better care quality, more efficient processes, and enhance the patient and staff satisfaction.

Governments or investors which having ageing hospital facilities may have to decide whether to renovate the building or build a new structure. Constructing a new building is the easiest way to embed all of the digital component shared in this chapter. Integration the hospital-of-the-future concept to a renovation project of archaic premises is more difficult. Unfortunately, for some facilities build something new is not an option; they should consider renovation with futuristic elements based planning.

It is possible that patient satisfaction has become a greater focus in the future hospitals, which is impacting the design and use of healthcare infrastructure outside of building codes or design standards. The investors', healthcare professionals' and patients' objectives and expectations from hospitals are evolved over the years. Taking account of these groups' considerations may provide further clues for future hospitals design.

No matter how it is done, a comprehensive digital strategy is required to create the hospital of the future. Some hospitals, keeping their operations away from technological advances and new economic trends with some reason. However, over time, they may experience challenges with the return on their investments.

Instead, the public or private hospital investors should consider investing digital building, creating an enterprise-wide digital strategy and linking this strategy into their processes.

Desired Outcome	EDB Recommendations
Reduction of Errors	Identical rooms
	Lighting
Incereasing Safety and Security	No slippery floors
	Appropriate door openings
	Correct placement of rails and accessories
	Correct toilet and furniture heaiht
	Single-bed rooms
	Easy-to-clean surfaces
	Automated sinks
	Smooth edges in rooms
Enhancing Control	Control over bed position
	Control over air temperature
	Control over lights
	Control over sound
	Control over natural light
Privacy	Single-bed rooms
	Design of waiting rooms
Comfort	Single-bed rooms
	Materials without glare
	Windows with a view
	Daylight
	Wayfinding

Table 2 - Desired Evidence-Based Design Outcomes and Recommendations
Adobtepd from Huisman et al

In order to best evaluate the use of Evidence-Based Design (EBD)

in healthcare renovation projects, it is first helpful to have an understanding of a few key elements. First, some high-level healthcare facility statistics and trends will be shared. The body of knowledge supporting EBD principles, as evidenced by the systematic reviews, is substantial enough to merit industry adoption and standardization. The list of EBD recommendations from the Huisman study are shown in Table 2, organized by the desired outcome each recommendation seeks to achieve.

When we look at the table, we see that 22 recommendation topics have been identified under 5 headings in the thesis of Whitaker. Almost all of these suggestions will the headings to be fulfilled during the digitalization process.

The increasing prevalence of chronic illness and an ageing population are pushing hospitals to pursue models of care that would best meet the needs of changing patients' demands across the care continuum. In this, hospitals should be ideally designed to lead and to create a true "system" of care delivery.

The implementation of digital technologies is already expanding the reach of hospital care into the community and into the home. Probably, the hospitals of the future will be defined by its intellectual property, rather than its physical facilities.
The physical design of the hospital together with its "digitalization" will have remarkable implications for the capability of the hospital to full fill its investment objectives for patient-centred care with clinically effective and collaboratively delivered services.

There are factors that will be different extents out of the hospital's control as the future unfolds. Hospitals need fair and rational payment strategies that align with national quality goals, but today's reality these cannot be assured. In the meantime, hospitals must increase efficiencies as a means of improving safety and decreasing costs. Digitalization can help to hospital for these kinds of objectives. The principles put forth in this chapter are intended to guide the hospitals, investors and governments to be better prepared to the hospital of the future and accomplish what is being expected of them.

Digital hospitals increase the speed and efficiency in administrative processes and cut the paper and document costs to zero. Diagnosis and treatment processes can be managed not only within the hospital walls but also from a distant location. Some follow-up processes can be managed by AI-technologies with sensors, cameras and early warning systems etc.

Digital integration at the point of care offers many advantages for the hospital and its patients. In the near future, digital hospitals will offer the most effective and efficient healthcare services to the patients within the shortest time.

As the final words; "The evidence-based list of recommendations suggests that future hospitals should be designed to work with digital technologies with the help of digital technologies".

References

1. Becker's Healthcare; "34 most expensive hospital expansion, renovation projects of 2016,", January 10, 2017. https://www.beckershospitalreview.com/facilities-management/34-most-expensive-hospital-expansion-renovation-projects-of-2016.html , accessed June 2, 2019.

2. Deloitte; The hospital of the future; How digital technologies can change hospitals globally, https://www2.deloitte.com/global/en/pages/life-sciences-and-healthcare/articles/global-digital-hospital-of-the-future.html

3. Huisman, E. R. C. M., Morales, E., Van Hoof, J., & Kort, H. S. M. (2012). Healing environment: A review of the impact of physical environmental factors on users. Building and Environment, 58, 70-80.

4. Indian Brand Equity Foundation, "Healthcare Update," January 2017. https://www.ibef.org/download/Healthcare- January-2017.pdf, accessed May 27, 2019.

5. Karine Chevreul, Karen Berg Brigham, Isabelle Durand-Zaleski and Cristina Hernández-Quevedo, "France: Health system review. Health Systems in Transition," European Observatory on Health Systems and Policies, ISSN 1817— 6119 Vol. 17 No. 3(2015). http://www.euro.who.int/__data/assets/pdf_file/0011/297938/France-HiT.pdf, accessed June 8, 2019.

6. Ministry of Health of Turkey, Sözleşmesi İmzalanan Şehir Hastaneleri https://sygm.saglik.gov.tr/TR,33960/sehir-hastaneleri.html accessed June 8, 2019.

7. Orlando Arango, "EIB loan for The Royal London and Barts Hospitals," European Investment Bank, April 27, 2006. http://www.eib.org/infocentre/press/releases/all/2006/2006-041-eib-loan-for-the-royal-london-and-barts-hospitals. htm?f=search&media=search, accessed June 2, 2019.

8. Reuters, "China to boost beds, staff to handle healthcare strains," January 11, 2017. http://www.reuters.com/article/ us-china-health-idUSKBN14V034, accessed May 27, 2019.

9. Taskin Kilic; Digital Hospital; An Example Of Best Practice; International Journal of Health Science Research and Policy; Volume 1; Issue 2; 2016; p 52-58

10. The Joint Commission; Guiding Principles for the Development of the Hospital of the Future; 2008

11. Vest JR, Gamm LD; Health information exchange: persistent challenges and new strategies. J Am Med Inform Assoc. 2010 May-Jun; 17(3):288-94.

12. Whitaker, David S., "The Use of Evidence-Based Design in Hospital Renovation Projects" (2018). All Theses and Dissertations. 6692. https://scholarsarchive.byu.edu/etd/6692 accessed June 8, 2019.

13. Zhuang Y, Sheets L, Shae Z, Tsai JJP, Shyu CR. Applying Blockchain Technology for Health Information Exchange and Persistent Monitoring for Clinical Trials. AMIA Annu Symp Proc. 2018; 2018: 1167–1175.
Published 2018 Dec 5.

Chapter XVI

-

Digital health and the future of healthcare

by Dr. H. Omer TONTUS

Introduction to Digital Health

The main purpose of digital health is to promote living healthy for anyone, anywhere, at any ages. It is generally accepted that digital health has the potential to support health systems for health promotion and disease prevention, globally. In order to realize this potential, a sound strategy that combines financial, organizational, human and technological resources should be determined in efforts to develop digital health solutions.

The digital health is a dynamical process and evolving rapidly. It has irrevocably changed the way healthcare systems are managed and the provision of health services and continues to do so. As a matter of fact, even the nomenclature shows a continuous renewal. For example, in the last five years, we have seen the terms telemedicine, eHealth, medical informatics, health informatics, telehealth and mHealth every day in newspapers or on the Internet. Whatever the meaning of these terms is for the author, these ultimately form a concept of digital health in readers. These terms are samples which used to describe the application of ICTs to healthcare. Eventually, the term digital health began to be used to cover all previously used terms.

Changing from eHealth/mHealth to digital health puts more importance on digital tool users. Digital health includes an extensive range of smart-tools and connected devices being used, together with other innovative and progressively flourishing concepts as that of IoTs and the wider use of AI, big data and analytics.

Health systems and healthcare delivery in a global manner are threatened by the rise of noncommunicable diseases, healthcare workforce shortages, ageing populations, unplanned emergencies and infectious disease outbreaks. Proper administration and use of digital technologies will help to overcome some of these challenges.

After the first wave of eHealth applications in the late 1990s and early 2000s, a more integrated approach to ICT for healthcare provision and patient care was understood as necessary. In the early period of 21st century, the target was changed to the integration of digitally provided services to use data and resource more efficiently, prevent disintegration, and simplify information sharing for better and faster decision-making. As a result of this change effort, studies have started to standardize digital health policies and strategies which will be called as digitalization.

Successful implementation of digital health goes beyond just the use of ICT to improve processes to meet needs. It must also cover subjects such as scalability, replicability, interoperability, security and accessibility. In the end, digital health should benefit people in a reliable, fair and sustainable manner. There are many models of ICT applications that are known to be useful in some areas, but fail to achieve the desired goals or demonstrate the expected expansion. Among other challenges, ICT applications that fail to integrate with other digital initiatives are unlikely to survive.

The proof on the influence of digital health tools, policies and strategies on health systems and on an individual's health or public health is steadily being cumulated. This can be explained by the fact that digital health is still in its early onset10. It may take years to measure the impact of digital health technologies on health systems. It is evident that the reliable use of digital healthcare applications will be possible with long-term collected data-based analyzes. Therefore, criteria and metrics should be defined in order to evaluate and interpret the progress. Defining the criteria will provide a basic platform for the development, consistent progress and monitoring of digital health applications.

The surge of new digital technology tools and techniques offers new alternative options of interacting with individuals, peoples, families, institutions, healthcare facilities, offices, patients and healthcare professionals. However, it is necessary to guide individuals to the use of increasingly sophisticated programs. Measures should be taken against the misuse of the collected personal data and the information shared through digital tools should be reliable and accurate. Additionally, individuals may not be sensible for the potential misuse or malicious use of new tools. Therefore, they must be appropriately informed about the potential risks. These are clearly the duty of policy-makers and governments.

Digital Health as a Concept

While digital health is a simple concept, it's an expansive and emergent sector. It can be clarified as "using advanced technologies to help improve person's health and wellness". It can include many things from wearables to ingestible sensors, from mobile health applications to AI, from robotics caregiver to EHR. Digital transformation is a process which includes cultural change and disruptively innovative technologies. If digital health solutions are transformed into attitudes by the individual or implemented to the institutional processes by an organization, digitalization is mentioned. Digitalization involves more than just the use of an application or software for an enterprise process. A digitalized hospital can be considered as a paperless hospital in a sense and the digitalization of healthcare is a rapidly evolving movement.

There are many drivers for cognitive technologies in health and the most important is "data". Health-related data is predicted to be doubled approximately every 10 weeks by 2020. Every individual is already producing plenty of health data within a lifetime to fill more than a couple of hundred million books. Doctors and other professionals cannot keep up with the growing amount of data which will be available to them.

Additionally, there are increasing challenges in physicians "shortage and burnout". In practice, primary-care physicians are working an average of 11 hours a day, of which 6 hours are used to interact with the EHR. Social determinants of health are covering almost 70% of all health determinants. Markers such as where we live, what we eat, total time we exercise, our stress levels are very important factors for our overall health. All of these determinants can be monitored with the help of digital health technologies. AI enables physicians to analyze a large amount of clinical data, genetic data, and health data to find the best for every patient.

Are digital health solutions really important?

Digital health is a sector in sectors. It is directly related by computer sciences sector and the healthcare sector. The aims of the digital health industry are various and complex such as preventing disease, helping patients' monitorization, management of chronic diseases, decreasing the cost of healthcare services, and making personalized medicine.
What makes digital health interesting for the healthcare sector is that its goals could potentially stand to benefit both patients and health care providers. By collecting health-related data from the intensity of activities to glucose levels, from heart rhythm to blood pressure, digital technologies will help individuals to improve their life habits and staying healthy, and so need fewer call or visit to their doctors.

Digital health technologies could also help to "recognize new diseases" or "the follow-up period of current illness". Digital health technologies could help longer disease-free life by enabling doctors to take an early step when symptoms of the disease started. Digital health tools also help to improve life quality and cut the total expenses of healthcare.

Companies in the digital health sector

Most of the major technology companies such as Apple, Alphabet, Google, Samsung, Amazon, IBM are interested in digital health, with different pathways.

For example, Google has the most widespread and one of the most far-sighted, strategy. It has solutions in the wearables market to track health data, over Google Wear, and Fit, since 2014.

However, it's putting effort into AI for healthcare with its DeepMind unit. Elsewhere, Alphabet has its health sciences unit, Verily. It is dedicated to using technology to understanding health better, as well as preventing, detecting, and managing the disease. Alphabet has a number of different ongoing health projects such as another health unit, Calico which has the task of "combating ageing". Calico is an R&D company with the mission of applying advanced technologies to promote our understanding of the biology of ageing for enabling people to lead longer and healthier lives.

In the present, Apple's strategy is creating an environment from the care provider to the individuals. In recent models, the functionality of the Apple Watch amplified for making it more health-focused with the "ECG monitoring" and "falls detection" specifications. These kinds of changes are laying the foundation for health provider companies to subsidize the Apple Watch for their patients and expand Apple's share of the wearables market. As one of the most powerful technology companies, Amazon has already bought a medication delivery company and entered the digital healthcare sector. Amazon plans to remake how healthcare is delivered in the USA, by forming its own health benefits platform.

IBM also engaging with the future of healthcare technologies. Watson is IBM's big plan on AI, and healthcare is a prime domain for IBM's present and future applications. Watson Health created for solving some of the world's most critical health problems thru data analytics and AI. By the combination of healthcare experts' opinions with augmented AI, Watson helps professionals and researchers around the globe to render data and transfer knowledge to make more informed decisions about treatment for their patients. There are expanding body of evidence backing Watson in healthcare. Watson Health has a distinctive method for the implementation of data-driven technology in the market. There are 80 AI Services behind IBM Watson that patients and healthcare providers can access. Watson Health made important progress within 5 years. Today, it has more than 15,000 clients and partners. Also, it has over 50 peer-reviewed articles as scientific evidence about Watson Health's importance. Articles demonstrate how Watson Health's AI data and analytic tools are being used in healthcare and life sciences. IBM has received or applied for more than 2,500 patents in health and life sciences in the US, 400 of which are unique to Watson Health.

One of the other application in the market is Zocdoc, which is backed by some of the biggest names in tech, such as Bezos, Benioff and Thiel's Founders Fund, is the latest highly-valued software start-up that's found it difficult to find sustainable growth in health care. It is an online medical care appointment booking service that provides free medical care search for end users by bringing together information about medical practices and personal schedules of doctors in a central location. By 2019, it has been expanded to cover 40% of the US population in more than 2000 cities and is used by more than 5,000,000 people monthly.

The key technologies that will shape the digital health market.

The user side of digital healthcare has been largely pushed by the advancement of wearable products and mobile healthcare applications. The explosion of digital health began with the presentation of wearables technologies such as FitBit wrist bands, the Apple Smartwatch and Samsung Galaxy Watch. In the very first years, consumers easily gathered data on their daily activity intensities, such as the number of steps, walking distance and minutes of physical activity. The mobile application ecosystem grew up around these kinds of gadgets and extended the ways that data could be analyzed and viewed.

Through apps, people learned that they can store, compare and share some of their health and health-related measurements. This has made people more demanding about digital health solutions. Thus, applications creators and hardware companies started expanding the range of apps and tools which help people to monitor their health-related data from heart rhythm to reproductive health. At least the first decade, most applications and equipment have focused on healthy lifestyle measures. This approach has changed. Applications and equipment are becoming more medical with sophisticated sensors and AI-techs. They inform individuals and physicians about glucose level, blood pressure, heart rate, and medications and drug side effects.

What problems do digital healthcare companies solve?

When applications and tools began collecting health data of individuals, it was only a matter of time before companies decided to see how they could derive money from them and this motive opened the new era for digital health.

There are many reasons why technology companies targeted the health sector in particular. One of them is that people want to know more about their health and the other one is that governments and investors target for reducing health expenses. These two headings pave the way for technology companies to develop new applications and intelligent technologies. Since the most important way to reduce the cost of health care is to do preventive medicine studies, this demand of the governments is tried to meet with the many different software prepared.

Many increasing diseases, such as type II diabetes, hypertension and high cholesterol level can be prevented or controlled by healthy lifestyle choices. This is where digital tools are located in. Digital healthcare equipment and applications can provide health monitorization and help individual to better address their health.

Trends and opportunities in digital health

Digital health is not just for 'lifestyle support' which can help developing an ecosystem. Individuals with chronic diseases can monitor and manage their health conditions. While digital health technologies give people the tools for a better lifestyle with the help of a smartphone and applications, adding AI-technologies can improve the medical management of disease, too.

For example, how can digital health technologies help a patient with diabetes: With a wearable device that automatically measures the patient's blood sugar level, the patient is informed of his or her clinical condition. Accordingly, with the help of the respective applications, the diet program can be reviewed and the AI integrated device according to the blood sugar level can provide the necessary insulin injection to the patient. In addition, if the blood sugar level is above or below the safe limits, it may send a warning signal to the patient's physician. While digital health would be keeping people healthier for longer, the final aim of using digital health technologies is to manage chronic diseases for cutting healthcare cost and reducing the burden of out-of-pocket payments by reducing the number of outpatient appointments, hospital admissions and ER visits etc.

While digital health technology manufacturers develop solutions for individuals, they also provide solutions for healthcare providers and healthcare professionals. For example, the ECG application of Apple's work on "Apple Watch Series 4". That watch having additional electrodes built into the back of the watch, as well as electrical heart sensors in the watch's crown. This application can record heartbeat and rhythm by using the sensor and then check the recording for life-threatening atrial fibrillation. This feature could be extremely useful to not only the watch owner but their physicians too. Likewise, Medtronic has an application that lets individuals with internet-enabled pacemakers share heart data via their smartphone with their physician. This is a medical-grade application for professionals. Medtronic also created an app called The MyCareLink Smart Monitor for heart tool for individuals to stay linked to their physician. The MyCareLink Smart Monitor is a convenient way to send heart function monitoring device information remotely to physicians between visits or whenever patients are not feeling well. MyCareLink is an application prescribed by the patient's doctor. As a result, remote monitoring of pacemakers and other cardiac devices is now the standard of care. One of the most important telehealth company American Well announced their virtual care platform in Epic's App Orchard. The application allows physicians to embed video visits into their existing clinical workflows and launch video consultation with a patient by one click. These are mentioned as examples, there are many other in use applications created by different informatics companies.

Size of the digital health market

While most researchers agree that the digital health sector's economic size is around hundreds of billions of dollars worldwide, it is not easy to put forward a definite number for the size of the industry.

For the size of the digital health market; while, Global Market Insights, for example, says USD 504.4 billion by 2025, while Transparency Market Research foresees USD 536.6 Billion by 2025. However, these reports are focused solely on the digital technologies used by the healthcare industry, such as digital prescription, EHR/EMR, and telemedicine.

Statements that take into account individuals' digital healthcare spending are much harder to produce. According to Research and Markets' report on mobile health, the world mobile health market will reach around $ 189 billion by 2025 which means 32.3% grow at CAGR. This forecast different than others it only takes into account mobile part of digital health technologies. Research and Markets' report's prediction is driven by the healthcare industry's interest in trimming costs by moving to "patient-centered care". The wearables health tools market is set to double in size between 2018–2022 as, according to CCS Insight research. They noted that shipments for wearable devices in 2018 was more than 115mn and will hit 233 million in 2022, increasing the market's value to over $25bn by the end of the forecast stage. CCS Insight stated that the growing market size would be driven by the massive demand for smartwatches, particularly. One of the most significant factors driving purchases of the wearables including smartwatches market is that wearables can be used "comfortably and practically" for tracking a person's health status. As stated by Research and Markets, the medical wearable devices market is expected to reach around $15bn by 2022, which means it will cover the big portion of the $27bn total market value which CCS Insight's prediction.

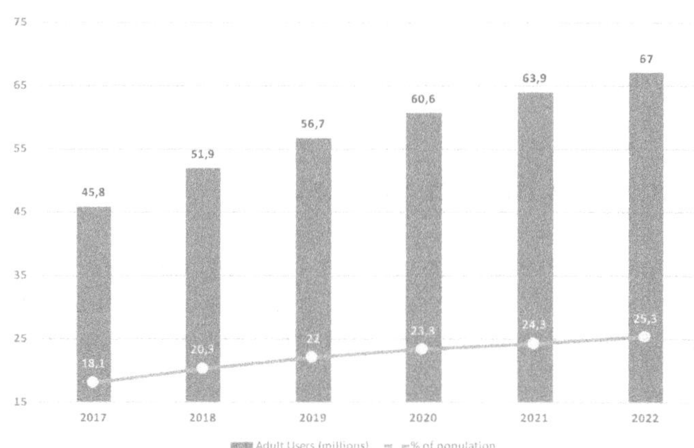

Graphic 6 - US Adult wearable users penetration data by years.
Adobtepd from eMarketer

	2019		2022	
	Wearable Users (millions)	**Internet User (%)**	**Wearable Users (millions)**	**Internet User (%)**
19-24	9,3	30,9	10,5	34,0
25-34	17,0	38,0	19,0	41,3
35-44	14,0	34,9	15,6	39,3
45-54	8,2	21,7	10,5	27,7
55-64	4,9	13,2	5,9	15,5
65+	3,3	8,6	4,7	10,9

Table 3 - Adult wearable users by age groups in 2019 & 2022.
Adobtepd from eMarketer

According on eMarketer data, in 2020, approximately 23% of US adults (almost 60 mn), will use a wearable gadget at least once a month, as shown in Graphic 6. Wearable technologies have attracted mainly to young and young-adult people. In 2015, 24.0% of those aged 25 to 34 had at least one wearables tool, while 6.5% of those aged 55 to 64 had one. In 2019, the 25-to-34 aged young adults will be the largest group of wearable users, with the highest penetration rate by jumping to 41.3%. But user penetration for the older people (55-64 years old) will also increase significantly to 15.5% as shown in Table 3. These figures are foreseen to increase in 2022. According to the eMarketer report, this increase is expected to be around 5% in the 18-54 age group.

Supplemental benefits of digital health

One of the most important gains of expanding the use of digital health technologies is creating and storing extensive data (big-data of healthcare) on health markers of individuals, all over the globe. In a couple of years, with the guidance of data mining and AI, researchers may be able to find the link between health issue and habits. In this way, researchers can determine the effect of whether or not to do something on the occurrence of a particular disease.
Concern for data security for an individual's sensitive health information exists in the healthcare industry, as in all other sectors. The data collected through digital technologies can provide a lot of important pieces of information for public health researches if used correctly.

Sample studies which conducted with help of digital health technologies

Smartwatches have the potential to support health in daily life by facilitating self-monitoring of personal activities, taking measures-based feedback, recognising individual behavioral patterns of surveys, and supporting two-way communication with doctors and relatives.

Stanford University conducted a clinical trial with more than 400,000 participants to identify whether a smartwatches application which analyzes heart-rate data can detect atrial fibrillation (AF) which is characterized by an irregular heartbeat. The results are published in November 2018 in the American Heart Journal. This was the most extensive screening research on AF has been ever done. Every year in the USA, atrial fibrillation causes more than 125,000 deaths and around 750,000 hospitalizations, according to the CDC. Each participant in the trial was required to have an Apple Watch and an iPhone. An application on the smartphone recurrently checked the heart-rate sensor to measure of an irregular pulse. The participants with recorded irregular pulse rhythm sections were sent a warning message and asked to visit a doctor in the study group. Participants with the irregular rhythm were then sent ECG to record the heart rhythm for up to a week. This clinical study probably will give first scientific proof for the capability of smartwatches algorithm to identify pulse irregularity and variability which may represent previously occult atrial fibrillation. The Apple Heart Study will help to maintain a basis for how wearable technologies can inform the clinical approach to AF diagnose and screening. These Stanford's study will also evaluate the practicability and scalability of pragmatic clinical studies using virtual and telemedicine studies designs. This important study results probably will support the importance of digital health technologies in the future and their inevitable use.

Another important literature example regarding smartwatch use has been published in the Journal of Pediatrics and Neonatology. Researchers used the smartwatch as a heart rate monitor in a preterm neonatal baby. As known, evaluation of the initial heart rate of a newborn after birth is the essence for deciding neonatal resuscitation. Before and during resuscitation the use three-lead electrocardiography recommended. But, the ECG monitors could be costly and is not exist in each delivery rooms. In their study, they used a smartwatch (Apple Watch 2) to detect the heart rate of a cyanotic preterm infant. They also used ECG monitor and oximetry simultaneously as control tools. A few seconds after implantation in the neonatal baby's chest wall, the smartwatch showed the same heart rate patterns with the ECG. At the end of the study, the researchers concluded that a smartwatch can be used as safely as ECG and oximeter even in preterm infants. The results of the similar AF trial study of University Hospital Basel is published in JACC: Clinical Electrophysiology journal. Trial results indicate that detection of atrial fibrillation by a smartwatch is in principally feasible, with very high diagnostic accuracy.

There are many articles published with the results of the studies conducted with Watson Health, IBM. Most of them related to oncological researches. For example, the "Manipal Comprehensive Cancer Center" study examined how "augmented AI" can assist breast cancer oncologists in clinical decision-making which published on "Annals of Oncolgy". Recommended therapies by "Watson for Oncology (WFO) and tumour board" for 638 breast cancer patients have compared. As a result, the treatment concordance rate between Watson health and the tumour board found in 93% of breast cancer patients. This study demonstrated that as the AI clinical decision-support system WFO can be a very helpful tool for breast cancer treatment decision making, especially at centres where breast cancer oncologists are limited.

Concerns over digital health

To better understand digital health and its contribution, it is necessary to ensure that it is used by a wide range of people and to assess its additive to individuals or institutions through user statistics. With this data, the contribution of digital health solutions to society and the health system can be analyzed. However, when we look at the users' demographic data, especially for wearable digital health devices, groups between the ages of 20-40 and middle-high income level appear. Therefore, it can be assumed that the usage data of digital tools do not provide information to evaluate the whole population.

For digital health products to contribute more to health professionals, they need to become more medicalised with technological advances and AI. Without AI support in the background and final assessments by health professionals, it is currently not appropriate to make an accurate diagnose or plan treatment with digital health technologies. Similarly, in smartwatches or fitness equipment groups, it's not really a clinical assessment that devices tell people they're good. If necessary, they can prevent the individual from going to the doctor.

Not only individuals or health care providers, but also insurers and government agencies have had to participate in the use of digital health in some way. For example, in Turkey, the Ministry of Health distributed 5 million units of free pedometer to combat obesity and promote a more mobile lifestyle, in the years 2013-2014. Similarly, lower insurance premiums may develop as an option for those who prefer healthy living and who have a low risk of unexpected illness and who are being followed up with digital health technologies. Some insurance companies encourage their customers to achieve healthy habits by offering discounted or free wearable products to customers who achieve certain exercise goals. It is not difficult to predict that data from such devices may one day affect pricing in health insurance policies. As a matter of fact, those who have an accident-free 5-year insurance history can get a discount on the price of car insurance up to 20% in the UK. Likewise, it is natural to expect a discount on health insurance policies for people who have a healthy lifestyle and who can be followed with digital technologies.

Final words

As a result, predicting that digital health technologies, especially smartwatches, will be used more extensively in the future does not require a wizard. The important aim of inventing more advanced digital technologies is to maximize its contribution to reducing governments' healthcare spending, prolonging individuals' disease-free survival, reducing insurance payments and providing better healthcare. The extensive range of digital health technologies includes many categories from health information technology to IoMT, from mobile health or wearables to telemedicine/telehealth and personalised medicine. Individuals and all other parties use digital health in efforts for decreasing inefficiency, lowering costs, improving access, and increasing quality.

The use of new technological advancements such as digital tools, social media, smartphones, wearables, IoT, IoMT and more others are changing the peoples' communication methods. But these kinds of innovations also providing better ways of monitoring health and well-being and offering superior access to informative data. Advances in digital health have led to the integration of information, technology, people and connections to improve health outcomes and health care.

References

1. Blaine Reeder, Alexandria David; Health at hand: A systematic review of smart watch uses for health and wellness; Journal of Biomedical Informatics; Volume 63, October 2016, Pages 269-276

2. Caitlin Stanway-Williams, Surging digital health market driving wearables market; October 2018, https://channels.theinnovationenterprise.com/articles/surging-digital-health-market-driving-wearables-market

3. Digital Health: Improving Lives; https://pharmeasy.in/blog/digital-health-improving-lives/

4. Digital Health Market will Reach USD 536.6 Billion by 2025 - Transparency Market Research September 2017, https://www.globenewswire.com/news-release/2017/09/22/1131466/0/en/Digital-Health-Market-will-Reach-USD-536-6-Billion-by-2025-Transparency-Market-Research.html

5. Global Digital Healthcare Market size to exceed $504.4 Bn by 2025 February 2019, https://www.gminsights.com/pressrelease/digital-health-market

6. Global $189 Billion Mobile Health Market, 2025; October 2017, https://www.prnewswire.com/news-releases/global-189-billion-mobile-health-market-2025-300535596.html

7. Jo Best; What is digital health? Everything you need to know about the future of healthcare; February 1, 2019 https://www.zdnet.com/article/what-is-digital-health/

8. Mintu P.Turakhia, ManishaDesai, HaleyHedlin, AmolRajmane, NishaTalati et al Rationale and design of a large-scale, app-based study to identify cardiac arrhythmias using a smartwatch: The Apple Heart Study; American Heart Journal Volume 207, January 2019, Pages 66-75 https://www.sciencedirect.com/science/article/pii/S0002870318302710?via%3Dihub

9. Marcus Dörr, Vivien Nohturfft, Noé Brasier, Emil Bosshard, Aleksandar Djurdjevic, Stefan Gross, Christina J.Raichle, Mattias Rhinisperger, Raphael Stöckli, Jens Eckstein; The WATCH AF Trial: SmartWATCHes for Detection of Atrial Fibrillation; JACC: Clinical Electrophysiology; Volume 5, Issue 2, February 2019, Pages 199-208

10. S. P. Somashekhar, M -J Sepúlveda, S Puglielli, A D Norden, E H Shortliffe, C Rohit Kumar, A Rauthan, N Arun Kumar, P Patil, K Rhee, Y Ramya, Watson for Oncology and breast cancer treatment recommendations: agreement with an expert multidisciplinary tumor board, Annals of Oncology, Volume 29, Issue 2, February 2018, Pages 418–423, https://doi.org/10.1093/annonc/mdx781

11. Stanford, Apple describe heart study with over 400,000 participants; https://med.stanford.edu/news/all-news/2018/11/stanford-apple-describe-heart-study-with-over-400000-participants.html

12. Watson Health: get the facts; November 2018, https://www.ibm.com/blogs/watson-health/watson-health-get-facts/

13. Wearables 2019, Advanced Wearables Pick Up Pace as Fitness Trackers Slow; January 2019, https://www.emarketer.com/content/wearables-2019

14. WHO (2018); Digital health; Seventy-First World Health Assembly; A71/A/CONF./1 Agenda item 12.4; 21 May 2018 http://apps.who.int/gb/ebwha/pdf_files/WHA71/A71_ACONF1-en.pdf

15. WHO/ITU National eHealth Strategy Toolkit, 2012, https://www.itu.int/dms_pub/itu-d/opb/str/D-STR-E_HEALTH.05-2012-PDF-E.pdf

16. WHO Global Strategy on Digital Health 2020-2024; 26 March 2019; https://extranet.who.int/dataform/upload/surveys/183439/files/Draft%20Global%20Strategy%20on%20Digital%20Health.pdf

17. Yung-Chieh Lin, Kai-Che Wei; An electronic smart watch monitors heart rate of an extremely preterm baby; Pediatrics & Neonatology Volume 59, Issue 2, April 2018, Pages 214-215

Chapter XVII

-

Driving forces and factors for the next generation hospitals

by Dr. H. Omer TONTUS

Hospital-based healthcare delivery is radically evolving in basic. Expectations of health service delivery and rapid technological transformations as well as structural changes force hospitals to produce new solutions. While the private health sector is strengthening in almost all countries, the existing hospitals somehow unite and form groups. Even the public sector concentrates its hospitals in certain centres. Independent large hospitals, once considered health care flagships, are no longer able to meet today's health needs. The latest example of health facilities that are structured in various corners of the city as seen in Ankara, Turkey's capital, each with 3000 beds vicinity is combined in two different health centre. In this way, the government predicted that it would save a significant amount of both personnel and other expenses. It also aimed to position experts from different hospitals in a well-known centre. Even if there are ideas that these projects will lead to urban patient mobility, the concentration of people in hospitals, traffic and parking problems, these huge complexes will need to be monitored for 2 years.

Both private and public hospitals should be structurally tailored to meet future needs and re-planning from supply chain to personnel management in all dimensions. Many external driving factors are affecting and will affect the work of hospitals. Whilst their relative importance differs from region to region, these factors are at play a role across the world. The followings are some of the most prominent driving factors of change in the literature.

Increase in chronic illnesses: The population is ageing and their aged peoples need are becoming more complex. The proportion of patients with more than one chronic diseases such as hypertension and diabetes mellitus is increasing. The expenses of caring for individuals with a long-term chronic illness is up to eight times higher than the caring cost of healthy adults. More people than ever before have survived after heart attacks and strokes within the last decades as a result of better care. These patients require significant post-hospital care need support to perform daily activities. The JAMA study found that diabetes was the medical condition responsible for the largest increase in expenditure during the study period when each disease separately analyzed. Following diabetes, top 5 conditions with the greatest increase in costs were low-back and neck pain, hypertension, high cholesterol level, depression and falls. According to the CDC, about 40% of American peoples are obese. This is of serious concern because obesity is causing a range of different important costly diseases. By contrast, only 4% of Japanese citizens are overweight. Obesity one of the most important chronic health problem of the US.

Population-related problems: On the one hand, the need to provide more health services due to population growth, on the other hand, increasing the elderly population leads to more costly health care. Therefore, almost 50% of the burden in health care expenditure comes from increased service costs, especially sharply rising inpatient services. Demographic trends in patient populations and increased cost of health care services are an important economic burden for both developed and developing countries.

As can be seen from Table 4, the US population increased by 9.5% from 2002 to 2009 and 7.5% from 2009 to 2016. From 2002 to 2016, there was a 17.6% population increase. However, the increase in the elderly population (over 65 years) was 17.1%, 22.4% and 43.3%, respectively. In other words, from 2002 to 2016, the elderly population growth rate is more than twice the general population growth rate. While the increase in per capita health expenditures in the general population was 207% from 2002 to 2016, this increase was even lower in the elderly population and became 191.6%. Due to the relatively rapid ageing of the population, the cost of the over 65 age group to the American economy increased by 274.6%. The healthcare expenditures of the elderly population, which was around 300 billion dollars in 2002, exceeded 825 billion dollars in 2016.

These figures show that the population is rapidly ageing and the increasing elderly population causes more health expenditure. Since the increase in the rate of the elderly population cannot be stopped, individuals should be given the habit of choosing a healthy lifestyle and should be protected from chronic diseases.

		2002	2009	2016	2002-2009	2009-2016	2002-2016
COST PER CAPITA	Total	3.345	4.810	6.929	143,8%	144,1%	207,1%
	Under 65	2.635	3.733	5.310	141,7%	142,2%	201,5%
	Over 65	8.275	11.716	15.851	141,6%	135,3%	191,6%
POPULATION	Total	288.181.763	315.465.351	338.971.420	109,5%	107,5%	117,6%
	Under 65	251.862.440	272.922.395	286.909.381	108,4%	105,1%	113,9%
	Over 65	36.319.323	42.542.956	52.062.039	117,1%	122,4%	143,3%
	% Over 65	12,6%	13,5%	15,4%			
TOTAL SPENDING (million)	Total	963.968	1.517.388	2.348.733	157,4%	154,8%	243,7%
	Under 65	663.658	1.018.819	1.523.489	153,5%	149,5%	229,6%
	Over 65	300.542	498.433	825.235	165,8%	165,6%	274,6%

Table 4 - Health care spending by year and age.

Expectation changes: Patients' and relatives' expectations are higher than ever before. Patients along with their relatives or caregivers look forward to receiving more detailed instruction about their situations, newest treatment options, and better amenities including medical tourism.8 They also want greater involvement in healthcare decisions and have higher standards. In addition, patients want to be more involved in health decisions about themselves. Patients want to make sure that customized and personalized solutions are produced as a result of easier access to information through digital technologies. Such a situation paves the way for the development of health models that prioritize patient comfort and satisfaction.

Community setting care: Patients are now requesting the healthcare outside of the hospital setting, if possible, and benefiting more from the health care provided in this way. Well-planned primary preventive care for patients in need of regular care due to chronic illness decreases both the frequency of possible complications and the need for hospital care. Such planning provides significant cost cuts, especially for reimbursement agencies and governments. Developing medical technologies and new surgical techniques have led to a reduction in complication rates and early postoperative discharge. This enables patients to return to their daily lives as soon as possible, and as a result, patient satisfaction rates are positively affected. Additionally, with support of surgical advances (such as LASIC eye surgery and laparoscopic procedures) are opened a new era for a growing number of procedures in outpatient settings. Increased demand for ambulatory health care services and urgent care centres is reflected in the sectoral growth in many countries such as the UK, Australia, Turkey and the USA.

Procedures in Outpatient Clinics: Over the last four to five years, there is an upward trend in outpatient clinic treatment. Instead of inpatient hospital procedure, patients and physicians are preferring the benefits of timely treatment at specialist outpatient centers. Insurance companies or reimbursement institutions encourage patients to be treated in outpatient institutions rather than in hospitals. In addition, physicians are now planning treatment in such centers more often to avoid intensive patient load and long waiting times. More importantly, ambulatory surgery centers and other outpatient centers now offer specialized and focused services for better patient care. There are also many different treatment methods ranging from minimally invasive vascular procedures to complicated surgical procedures can be performed in these settings.

Need for specialized centers of excellence: The treatment success rate is increasing in centers where experienced specialists in a particular procedure are concentrated. In many countries, some centers are specialized in certain procedures such as prosthesis surgery, interventional radiology, laser eye surgery, and cancer surgery. As shown in many works of literature, patient satisfaction increases as well as the success of treatment in institutions where advanced areas such as stroke centers, organ transplantation centers, burn centers, oncology centers serve. These providers effectively disintermediate general hospitals as a place for the provision of some types of specialist care. Advanced specialization brings with it some problems. The problem of physicians' shortage deepens as the number of physicians who are turning towards branches requiring extreme expertise. Although the success rate of treatment increases, advanced research centers (or centers of excellence) increase the cost of medical treatment. This dilemma shows that governments and reimbursement institutions should seek a solution together in favor of the patient.

Higher quality and better outcomes with clinical advancement: Advancements in clinical knowledge have driven to some truly remarkable achievements. For example, although the burden and risk factors remain alarmingly high, from 2006 to 2016, the annual death rate attributable to coronary heart disease declined approximately 32% and the actual number of deaths declined around 15%, according to the American Heart Association. Similar decline have been observed in some other developed countries. The lower mortality is a result of better diagnosis techniques, better treatment options and a better understanding of the underlying risk factors. As a result of new therapy models decrease in mortality from breast cancer and prostatic cancer are also striking. For many patients, advancement in antiretroviral drugs has converted AIDS from being a deadly disease to a chronic condition. The development of sofosbuvir for the treatment of chronic hepatitis C infection as a component of a combination antiviral treatment regimen has improved prognoses of hepatitis C patients. However, most of the clinical advances and new medications are at a very high cost. This results in devastating costs for reimbursement agencies, governments and out-of-pocket payers.

Digital technologies changed healthcare delivery: Digital health technologies are driving changes in care delivery, including remote access to EHR and AI. It is an expansive and emergent sector and includes many tools from wearables to applications, from AI to robotic surgery. Digital health technologies help to "diagnose diseases" or "the follow-up period of chronic condition". They also support longer disease-free life period by supporting doctors for an early step when symptoms of the disease noticed. Digital technologies also help to cut the total expenses of healthcare and free up time for staff to provide patient care. They also enable both patients and care professionals to play a major role through access to personal health data. AI implemented real-time management applications for decision support can reduce variability in the care type and improve the timing of care.

Unmanageable and worsening scarcity of healthcare professionals: It is known that there is approximately 7 million health workers' shortage in 2013 worldwide. This number is estimated to reach 13 million in 15 years. Shortage of caregivers are expected to increase pressure on the workforce, leading to overwork and burnout of employees. As such, children of health workers who see "the harsh working conditions and working hours" of their parents stay away from all types of the health sector workforce positions. For example, with exam result rankings based registration area college students about half of the students who rank first among 1,000 people in Turkey 10 years ago, medical schools prefer this ratio has now fallen to a tenth of a percentage. Also, it is more difficult, to attract students to nursing programs.

Difficult to finance healthcare: According to an article which focused on health care spending published in JAMA in 2017, there are 5 key factors associated with the rise of healthcare cost which are population growth, ageing, disease prevalence or incidence, medical service utilization and service price and intensity. The study indicated that healthcare service price and intensity, including the rising cost of pharmaceutical drugs, made up more than 50% of the increase.

The USA healthcare spending has been projected to exceed 24% of GDP by 2040. Reimbursement companies, insurers, employers and governments are struggling to find finance to keep up with the high yearly expansion of health care costs. Thus, they are putting more and more pressure on healthcare provider companies and caregivers (including nurses and physicians) to deliver affordable high-quality care. Finance needs are also an issue for the renovation projects of aged infrastructure and to invest for new technologies. Government programs (such as Medicare and Medicaid) increased demand for medical services, resulting in higher prices. Additionally, as mentioned above, increases in the incidence of chronic conditions like diabetes and heart disease are responsible for most of the healthcare costs and almost half of the all Americans have at least one chronic illness.

Soaring Health Insurance Premiums and Out-of-Pocket Payments: For almost all people, the rising price of health insurance premiums is at the centre of concerns about rising health care costs. In the US, the average annual premium for family healthcare coverage increased by about 5% in 2018, according to the National State Legislation Conference (NCSL). The two most-mentioned reasons for these increases were government policies and lifestyle habit changes. Higher insurance premiums are only part of the picture. Americans are paying more out-of-pocket than ever before. Middle-income families spend 11% of their incomes to out-of-pocket healthcare expenditures and insurance premiums and deductibles. A shift to high-deductible health plans can impose out-of-pocket costs increment.

Medical Tourism Realities: Medical tourism has become a popular way to dodge high healthcare costs and waiting lists in developed countries. In 2017, 1.4 million Americans travelled across the border to seek medical treatment as medical travellers. Since 2010, the number of Americans travelling cross-border for medical tourism has almost doubled.

The number of medical tourists to all countries in 2019 was estimated at over 16 million. The number of medical tourists in the world is expected to increase by 25% per year. The financial implications of medical tourism are also profound. The average cost for each medical visitor is on average $5,000 (1000-12,000) per visit, and in total yearly global estimation is at somewhere near $80 billion. Given the bigness of revenues related to medical tourism, it is not surprising that many countries such as India, Costa

Rica, Turkey and Malaysia actively focused on medical tourism. Facilitators like in conventional tourism are readily available all over the globe to help arrange admission to various hospitals and access to physicians throughout the world.

Patients Who Avoiding from Healthcare: Increasing healthcare service costs have generated an important problem. There are many people who afraid of the costs that will be billed by the healthcare providers. They escape any kind of medical care. A poll revealed that in 2017, 44% of Americans refused to go to a doctor due to cost concerns. 40% of them said they skipped a medical test or treatment within the last 12 months due to cost, and 32% were unable to fill a prescription because of its cost. 40% of them said they fear the costs associated with a serious illness, this number is more than who said they fear the illness itself. In many cases, those who refuse treatment even have medical insurance. Delaying treatment because of cost afraid eventually leads to even more costly health care services.

Healthcare Cyber-security issues: It is clear that healthcare institutions will take bigger steps in the near future better cyber-security standards like other industries. Health institutions are far behind the banking and retail sectors in terms of cybersecurity standards. Healthcare data is more valuable for cybercriminals from ant other sectors' data. The data held by health institutions includes not only credit card data but also sensitive data of the individual's whole life and of course it is more valuable. Healthcare institutions will invest more and more in IT security measures to protect data from cybercriminals.

Measuring quality metrics of healthcare: In the past, patients had limited data about the care quality of their hospitals and physicians. Today, hospitals in Scandinavia, Canada and the UK are legally pushed to publish quality measurements such as mortality rate, re-admittance rate and infectious complications rate, voluntarily sharing some additional metrics with the public. Furthermore, in many cases, financial bonuses are being awarded for the provision of high-quality care, especially in private practice hospitals. Performance-related payments are linked to quality targets and compliance with clinical guidance. In England, NHS providers have an incentive to support advancement in quality, they are given supplemental funds for delivering described improvements, as set out in the NHS standard contract. Hospitals should have unique quality elements to attract and retain both reimbursement institutions and patients. It has become a necessity to evaluate the information obtained through data analysis according to standard quality criteria and share it with the public.

Final words

The impact power of these factors may vary according to time and region and many different factors will rise and play a role in the sector. Health service delivery, which is a part of the service sector (according to WTO), is dependent on people as in other service sector sub-headings and it will continue to depend on the individual for many years. As a solution, healthcare providers develop and implement innovations on how to achieve better care. Hospitals use digital technologies to guide patients and make better agreements with reimbursement institutions. Better analyzed data provide information for hospitals to perfect themselves.

References:
1- American Heart Association Heart Disease and Stroke Statistics-2019 At-a-Glance; https://healthmetrics.heart.org/wp-content/uploads/2019/02/At-A-Glance-Heart-Disease-and-Stroke-Statistics-%E2%80%93-2019.pdf
2- Braverman B. 1.4 million Americans will go abroad for medical care this year. Should you? Available at: http://www.thefiscaltimes.com/2016/08/17/14-Million-Americans-Will-Go-Abroad-Medical-CareYear-Should-You. Accessed 11 June 2019.
3- Busse R et al. Tackling chronic disease in Europe: Strategies, interventions and challenges. European Observatory on Health Systems and Policies. 2010.
4- Dalen J.E., Alpert J.S., Medical Tourists: Incoming and Outgoing; The American Journal of Medicine, Jan 2019; Volume 132, Issue 1, 9 – 10
5- Dash P., Henricson C., Kumar P., Stern N.; The hospital is dead, long live the hospital!; Mc Kinsey & Company, May 2019; 2-18
6- Degala S., (2018); Five innovation trends that will impact the healthcare industry in 2018 https://medcitynews.com/2018/12/five-innovation-trends-that-will-impact-the-healthcare-industry-in-2019/?rf=1 Accessed on 11 June 2019
7- Dixon L. The state of the health care worker shortage. Talent Economy. November 17, 2017.
8- Edwards JD et al. Trends in long-term mortality and morbidity in patients with no early complications after stroke and transient ischaemic attack. Journal of Stroke and Cerebrovascular Disease.2017;26(7):1641–5.
9- Glenngård AH. The Swedish health care system. The Commonwealth Fund.

Accessed 3 June 2019.

10- Global Burden of Cardiovascular Diseases Collaboration. The Burden of Cardiovascular Diseases Among US States, 1990-2016. JAMA Cardiology. 2018; 3(5): 375–89.

11- Gonçalves-Bradley DC et al. Early discharge hospital at home. Cochrane Database of Systematic Reviews. 2017; 6: CD000356.

12- Heath S.; Insured Patients See High Premiums, Out-of-Pocket Healthcare Costs; December 2018; https://patientengagementhit.com/news/insured-patients-see-high-premiums-out-of-pocket-healthcare-costs

13- Jonkman NH et al. Do self-management interventions in COPD patients work and which patients benefit most? An individual patient data meta-analysis. International Journal of Chronic Obstructive Pulmonary Disease. 2016; 11: 2063–74.

14- NHS England. Commissioning for quality and innovation (CQUIN) guidance for 2017–2019. NHS publications gateway reference 07725. March 2018.

15- NORC at the University of Chicago & West Health Institute; Americans' Views Of Healthcare Costs, Coverage, And Policy; 2018; https://www.westhealth.org/wp-content/uploads/2018/03/WHI-Healthcare-Costs-Coverage-and-Policy-Issue-Brief.pdf

16- Patients Beyond Borders. Medical tourism statistics and facts. Available at: https://patientsbeyondborders.com/medical-tourism-statistics-facts Accessed 12 May 2019.

17- Probasco J., Why Do Healthcare Costs Keep Rising?, October 2018, https://www.investopedia.com/insurance/why-do-healthcare-costs-keep-rising/

18- Quinn TC. HIV epidemiology and the effects of antiviral therapy on long-term consequences. AIDS. 2008;22 (Suppl 3): S7–12.

19- Schmidt M et al. 25 year trends in first time hospitalisation for acute myocardial infarction, subsequent short and long term mortality, and the prognostic impact of sex and comorbidity: a Danish nationwide cohort study. BMJ. 2012;344:e356.

20- Varadarajan T. The business of saving lives. WSJ Opinion. October 20, 2017.

21- WHO Global health workforce shortage to reach 12.9 million in coming decades. World Health Organization. November 11, 2013.

Chapter XVIII

-

New Trends and Innovations in care delivery

by Dr. H. Omer TONTUS

According to some news headlines, robots and artificial intelligence (AI) will replace people as the workforce of the future. For example, an NBC headline says, "Will robots take your job? Humans ignore the coming AI revolution at their peril.", The New York Times writes, "Will robots take our children's jobs?". These stories portraying the future workforce. But the future for healthcare professionals might be much more optimistic. In Sarah Thomas opinion; "rather than replacing people in the healthcare workforce, technology could help healthcare institutions for creating more professionally satisfied employees at all levels".

An urgent in healthcare worldwide is improving quality and providing efficiency while controlling costs and expenditures. There is a tremendous diversity between hospitals, even between two hospitals of the same group, which results in remarkable differences in both the care quality and the care cost, worldwide. Hospitals and healthcare organizations are moving from being a service provider for patients. Surely, hospitals will provide health care to patients, but they also have to provide guidance to patients to protect their health and choose a healthy lifestyle. In basic, hospitals' architecture, the way they deliver health services, waiting rooms, processing times are changing to serve patients and health professionals successfully.

But more importantly, hospitals around the world are introducing new innovations for better care, day by day. Although these innovations have many different purposes for the healthcare providers, the following aims generally come to the fore: to strengthen clinical quality; to be personalized, focusing patient-centered care; improving patient experience; and increasing the productivity and efficiency. Each of these goals is an urgent necessity for today's hospitals.

Adopting lean processes

"Lean processes" encourage continuous improvement and is based on the idea of respect for people. Womack & Jones outlined the 5 principles of the lean process in their book. The five principles include;
> *1. Defining value,*
> *2. Mapping the value stream,*
> *3. Creating flow,*
> *4. Using a pull system,*
> *5. Pursuing perfection.*

Lean hospital management is based on insights from Lean management. "Lean process" or "Lean management" or only "Lean" for the hospitals is a set of operating philosophies and methods that help create maximum value for patients by reducing waste and waits. It improves hospitals profitability by reducing waste and improving patients' satisfaction. Lean healthcare in hospital is the application of "lean" ideas to care delivery facilities to minimize waste in every process, procedure, and task. Using lean principles, from physicians to administrative personnel all members of the institution have to be part of elimination anything that does not add value for patients.

Some of the hospitals are started to offer more successful services in terms of management and service delivery by eliminating waste with support for monitarization based on AI and the digital central control unit. These kinds of success stories are easily adapted by other hospitals with little differences.

As an example, the Beth Israel Medical Center has worked with data scientists from Amazon and Google to analyze seven petabytes of data to find tips and clues to better use healthcare resources while providing clinical care. With this kind of data analysis, AI can be used to increase the efficiency of the medical team by monitoring instant control of ambient temperature and ventilation during long operations. The Vall d'Hebron University Hospital provides another example of how the application of lean processes shapes clinical productivity. Operating theatres in the hospital are monitoring by a control unit that monitors the effective patient and staff movements as well as accelerating the supply of needed materials in the room.

Another important example is a study at the University of Pennsylvania Hospital (HUP), a 789-bed adult, acute care hospital. Continuous observations for safety precautions at HUP cost the hospital more than $1 million annually. In addition to the significant cost, safety precautions cause a resource strain when Clinical Nursing Assistants (CNAs) are pulled from daily care duties. HUP initiated a project to reduce the utilization of continuous observations and project is studied in a 116 beds part of the hospital. After analyzing the data, they determined that patients were remaining on continuous observation longer than clinically recommended. The HUP team developed a behavior tracking tool and a standardized process for reassessment. At the end of the initial project period, the results showed a nearly 5,000 hours waste of time in 12 months period in pilot units. At the end of the study, HUP found that the nurses which are important to increase patient satisfaction lost time in unnecessary duties. With the lean process management has enabled nurses to engage more with their actual tasks.

If lean healthcare is implemented correctly, it's an opportunity to better care service for patients and improve internal processes for hospitals. Many hospitals associate "lean" with cutting down resources or forcing employees to take on too much of a workload. Actually, the crucial idea behind "lean" is to improve efficiencies and provide high-quality care, by eliminating the waste processes that don't contribute to high-quality healthcare. That's an aim for every healthcare institutions. Lean is an innovative management strategy which has proven successful in healthcare institutions. It supports improving quality and efficiency while controlling costs for optimum patient care. Implementing the Lean is to manage difficult, everlasting continuous improvement processes. Lean convert the institutional culture from the inside out, with challenges and opportunities. It engages the entire staff in identifying and solving problems. The fundamental objective of Lean is to improve value for the patients and its tried methods came up with hope for higher quality healthcare at a lesser cost.

Professional staff problems

In response to the increasing cost and the worsening shortage of healthcare professionals, hospitals have started to change their organizational and managerial concept. Most of them are trying to free up the time of highly trained professional staff to perform activities for which particular high qualifications are critical. Many hospitals have expanded the use of trained technicians in healthcare services to assist specialist physicians. For example, in order to make more use of anesthesiologists, "anesthesia technicians" (or certified registered nurse anesthetists; CRNA) are working more often in the operating theatres. In routine procedures, the process other than the initial phase and wake-up phase of general anesthesia is carried out under the control of trained anesthesia technicians. In the USA anesthesia technicians (CRNA) administered anesthetics approximately more than 40 million times, in

2017. Another example is that India's Aravind Eye Hospital has expanded the use of technicians to help eye surgeons perform specific tasks during the operation in the purpose of to make eye surgeons more efficient by making more cases.

Some study reports have underlined the possibilities of technological solutions for some of the workforce shortages in healthcare delivery. For example, automation systems, digital technologies and AI can enable physicians and other healthcare professionals to get laboratory test results or radiological images faster and increase productivity by enabling them to focus more effectively on better patient experience. Automatons or robotics could also take roles in routine processes such as dispensing of prescribed drugs to the department.

Rapidly emerging digital technologies are driving increased automation which affecting the nature of work and workforce talent models. Many healthcare provider organizations are having problems with change and its implications on the workforce. These organizations need to keep in mind with changes "such as robotics, AI, digital tools" are the great opportunity to alleviate nursing shortages and physician burnout.

While industrial robots and automation systems are becoming more capable and less expensive every year, there are approximately 9 times more data circulation through business than two years ago and the half-life of a skill is now very short. Traditional employment has been replaced by a talent continuum which comprises not only full- and part-time workers, but also freelancers and automated labor. In healthcare, we can easily say that the workforce, digital technologies and well-developed robots will be integrated into the care delivery. Digital technology operated kiosques, movement detectors (such as fall detector), and voice recognition brought convenience to patients and healthcare organizations. In many hospitals, robots are assisting for logistic tasks such as distributing linens, meals, and medical supplies or collecting test samples or test results. Such technological advances have allowed staff to allocate more time to patient care. By integrating digital technology and AI across all operating systems of the hospitals improved physician and staff productivity can be obtained which will be resulted in increased quality in care delivery and improved patient and visitor experiences with better satisfaction.

Example of basic changes

• Blockchain also is started to transform health care. It can help institutions bridge traditional data which impressively increase IT and organizational performances, keep all data secure, and streamline patients' access to medical data. Blockchain offers "long data" as opposed to big data, capturing a full history of a patient's health.

• New diabetes drugs and advanced AI supported monitoring technologies will lower complications and make better the management of diabetes which could bring a shift in the medicines prescribed and ways of managing type 2 diabetes. Glucose sensing technologies are rapidly advancing, moving from low-tech finger pricks to continuously simultaneous glucose monitoring with a sensor which placed beneath the patient's skin.

• Drones also will play an increasingly prominent role in bringing medical care to patients in an emergency condition. It will help to connect remote communities to distant clinics. Drones will carry blood, vaccines, and other medical necessities and patient samples to and from regional hospitals.

• Use of point-of-care (POC) diagnostics will gain speed. The expanding of borderless hospitals and community care is increasing the need for rapid results outside of the clinical setting. The major key factor for the future of healthcare delivery is moving toward home health care.

• Demand for surgical, rehabilitation and hospital robots will continue to rise. Driven by declining costs and staff shortages, healthcare robots deployed in the years ahead will be involved in the surgery, in-hospital logistics, disinfection, caregiving, physical rehabilitation, and prosthetic limbs. Forecasts suggest that health care robot shipments will increase from approximately 3,400 sold annually in 2016, to more than 10,500 per year by 2021, representing an increase in revenues from $1.7 billion to well over $2.5 billion over the same time period.

Technological improvements in inpatient care

In 1988, When I was a resident in general surgery program there was 36 other residents beside me. I was given the task of scheduling night shifts for doctors in training and it was a disaster for me to schedule night shifts for each resident doctor every month. I hadn't been working as a doctor for days while planning with so many criteria like their competitors, diseases leave, wedding anniversaries, birthdays, colleagues who did not want to work together on shift. But, in today's practice, the AI technology based scheduling of patients' and personnel's time is a new normal. Probably it takes a couple of minutes to announce the work schedule of residents. Technology is already shaping the delivery of care in many hospitals. Hospitals have installed automation systems to help staff spend more time with patients and create a reliable care environment for patients.

Scheduling resources in an efficient and cost-effective way is challenging, and at many hospitals, these tasks are often left to individuals with limited training or experience. To solve this problem, a Massachusetts Institute of Technology (MIT) trained robot has learned to function as a nurse manager of sorts, making workflow suggestions in real time. This developed AI robot already works for automating hospital scheduling of physicians and other healthcare professionals. By 2025, according to the WEF, machines will do at least 50% of the workplace duties, this number is around 30% in today's world. This change will enable people to take responsibility for higher-level roles that require unique creativity, emotional intelligence and leadership. The developed AI assistant plans which room will be logistically more accurate for the hospitalized patient and can determine which nurse will more benefit to the patient according to the work experience. Moreover, the AI supported solutions create more equal workload, and could help improved staff satisfaction.

AI integrated decision support systems improve not only administrative processes but also patient follow-up procedures. During the monitoring of vital functions of the patients, AI-systems inform the nurses if the predefined limit values of the patients (such as pulse rate, blood glucose level, PaO2) are exceeded which provides better care quality.

With the evidence-based algorithms, clinicians can make a more accurate diagnosis and treatment decisions in favour of the patient. Radiodiagnostics using AI-enabled can open new dimensions to achieve better efficiency of radiologists and greater accessibility for clinicians.

With the assistance of digital technologies or smartphones applications, trained specialists can help to diagnose a pathology from any location of the globe using the imaging techniques from MRI to CT-Scan. This may contribute to reducing the shortage of specialist workforce opinion, which is seen as the biggest problem of health services in the future.

Software may help to doctor in diagnose, and that highly well-aimed technology may be available to both physicians and patients via smartphones. Many software companies and research teams are currently working to combine AI into medical education, training and practice via clinics, hospitals, universities and smartphones.

A research team at Stanford recently reported that their software had learned to classify skin cancer with a level of competence equivalent to that of board-certified dermatologists. Cutaneous cancer is one of the most common human malignancy which principally diagnosed by visual, clinical and dermoscopic analysis followed by a biopsy and histopathological evaluation. A research group from Stanford demonstrated classification of skin lesions using a single deep convolutional neural networks (CNNs), trained end-to-end from images directly, using only pixels and disease labels as inputs. They trained a CNN using a dataset of almost 130000 clinical images consisting of more than 2000 different diseases. Researchers tested its performance against 21 board-certified dermatologists on biopsy-proven clinical images and CNN achieved performance on par with all tested experts. The study demonstrated that AI is capable of classifying skin cancer with a level of competence comparable to dermatologists. Smartphones with deep neural networks can amplify the role of dermatologists and can provide low-cost global access to critical diagnostic care.

CellScope Oto is designed to allow physicians to easily take, view, store and share high-quality magnified images of the tympanic membrane. When used with a custom mobile phone application, it offers an option to take digital ear exams wirelessly. The CellScope Oto is clinically validated by hospitals and providers across the US. Two different clinical studies prove that the use of smartphone-enabled otoscopes, such as the CellScope, has the potential to improve patient care. One study result is from Neurotrauma Center at University of California Irvine School of Medicine, Irvine Medical Center which included neurotrauma patients. Another study result is from Emory University, Atlanta which included pediatric Otitis Media patients. Both are agreed that the use of smartphone-enabled otoscopes, such as the CellScope, has the potential to improve patient care.

Some examples of medical applications are functional both for the physicians and the people.

• PEPID Knowledge Base: It is an important developer of clinical and drug information resources and mobile apps for healthcare providers, hospitals and medical faculties. PEPID gives access to disease data, drugs info, drug interactions and side effects, drug details, and it can use data directly from institutions' EMR, EHR, ePrescribe, or other healthcare information system.

• UpToDate: It is an application from Wolters Kluwer for clinical decision support and linked with better patients' outcomes. More than 1.7 million physicians globally use UpToDate for making better care decisions. There are almost 100 research studies which demonstrate its impact on better patient care and hospital performance, including decreased lengths of hospital stay, fewer adverse effects, and lower mortality. These impacts can lead to significant savings for organizations.

• Lippincott Advisor: It delivers evidence-based practice information that is specifically designed to give immediate access to the clinical answers for physicians need at the point-of-care. It is a web-based application which has the ability to integrate directly into the EMR. It provides direct information on diseases, diagnostic tests, drugs, treatments, signs & symptoms, care plans, guidelines etc.

• ScienceSoft company providing hospitals, ancillary providers and assisted living organizations with operational technology and electronic health record solutions to collect, process and analyze clinical data including patient, treatment and medication information. The software is helping the caregivers track patients' health status during their stay by the health monitoring module functionality on two groups (vitals and test results). The vitals module includes data such as BP, pulse rate, respiration rate, body temperature, weight, height, BMI. The test results module includes records on blood glucose level, INR level and pulse oximetry.

Effect of Innovations to Treatment

Innovations in medical treatment have an important effect on the expanding of treated disease and individuals. Both the changes in the pharmacological field and the new options developed in the treatment protocols reflected as the increasing cost to health systems.

Below are some examples of innovatively developed treatment modalities:

• **Stem cell therapy:** According to the FDA, stem cell therapies may offer the potential to treat for few diseases or conditions. Sometimes called the body's "master cells," stem cells are the cells that develop into blood, brain, bones, and all of the body's organs. They have the potential to repair, restore, replace, and regenerate cells, and could possibly be used to treat many medical conditions and diseases. Today, physicians routinely use stem cells that come from bone marrow or blood in transplant procedures to treat patients with cancer and disorders of the blood and immune system. As stated by CBC Canada, the cost of stem cell therapy is $5,000 to $8,000 per stem cell treatment for patients. According to a Twitter poll by BioInformant, the cost can be even higher, with stem cell treatments costing as much as $25,000 or more. For treatments that require a systemic or whole-body approach for complex diseases such as Crohn's disease and multiple sclerosis, the cost tends to be in the higher range, often averaging from $20,000 to $30,000.

• **Innovative cancer treatments:** Conventional therapies for cancer such as surgical procedures, chemotherapy and radiotherapy remain a mainstay in treatment. However, in some cases, a classically targeted treatment approach is not enough for expected outcome and patients may be vulnerable to drug resistance. In recent years, new concepts are emerging to improve traditional treatment options for cancers with poor survival outcomes. New therapeutic strategies, including advances in nanotechnology and immunotherapy involving areas such as energy metabolism and extracellular vesicles, guide new generation cancer therapies. The development of areas such as theranostics in nanomedicine opens new doors for targeted drug delivery and nano-imaging. Smart and highly engineered nanoparticles give great advantages for targeting drugs to specific cells or tissues, with high solubility, bioavailability, biocompatibility, and multifunctionality. As another innovative therapy, targeting cancer cells selectively through their mitochondrial defects have been shown to augment the anti-tumor effects of treatment. Drugs which target regulate mitochondria function and metabolism and simultaneously increase sensitivity to induction of apoptosis may be the most effective anti-cancer agents. Some examples of the innovative cancer therapies include gene therapy, laser therapy, nanotechnology and nanoparticles, RNA interference therapy, photosensitizer and hyperthermia.

• **Implantable cardioverter defibrillators (ICDs):** It is a device which implantable inside the body, able to perform cardioversion, defibrillation, and pacing of the heart. Studies have shown ICDs are effective in preventing sudden death or cardiac arrest in high-risk patients, sustained life-threatening ventricular arrhythmias. Newest ICDs also have a dual function which includes the ability to serve as a pacemaker. Implantable string subcutaneous defibrillator (ISSD) can be accepted as the newest generation ICDs. It has been designed to be placed without the need for a surgical pocket, may allow improved patient conformity and aesthetics. Also, it is less invasive with optimal only 20 minutes of implantation time. Unlike commonly used ICDs, the ISSD doesn't require a metal pulse generator pocket. Instead, it uses a single flexible string-shaped device with no leads within the heart. ISSD can be connected to a smartphone. The ICD costs include device and implantation, as well as costs for follow-up. The ICD costs cover an ICD lifetime of 6 years. On a per-day basis, ICDs are more expensive than ACE-inhibitors, statins, and beta-blockers.

• **Robotic sleeve:** Harvard University researchers alongside with Boston Children's Hospital researchers have produced (or invented) a personalized soft robot (or robotic hand-like device) that covers around the heart and helps it beats, potentially opening new treatment options for patients with heart failure. The Robotic sleeve promises great hope for patients who have a heart attack with a weakened heart and are at risk for heart failure. The robot syncronizes with the patient's heart through a thin silicone sleeve with soft pneumatic actuators that imitate the heart's muscle. It provides ventricular assistance without blood contact. This removes the need for anticoagulant medications.

• **3D bioprinted tissue:** 3D bio-printing is a technological advancement which opened an era that enables fabrication of biomimetic, multiscale, multi-cellular tissues. It gives the option to produce the tissue-specific composition. Although there is an increasing demand for organ transplants, the number of organ donors is limited. Therefore, bioprinting is a potential technology that can solve the crisis of organ scarcity by fully functional organ production. The entire process is highly complex. It involves re-programing a patient's blood cells into stem cells, which are then mutated to produce the specific types of cells suitable for the 3D bioengineering.

• **Precision Medicine:** The rise of precision medicine or pharmacogenomics will significantly influence pharmaceutical research and healthcare technology. This approach has achieved great success in oncologic therapy by focusing on the genetics of the patient in order to offer better treatment prescriptions for patients. By decoding the genetic profiles of patients' tumours, oncologists can decide which treatments will work best for which patients.

Technology-assisted healthcare at the outside of the hospital

Technology improves and supports remote care for "better patient experience and patient satisfaction", as a result of provided higher clinical quality. In the near future, many clinical healthcare services will likely move to remote mode of cares by the help of telemedicine and real-time or on-demand consultations. Hospitals can reduce their costs whilst providing healthcare to people by using digital, robotics and AI technologies. Remotely accessible technologies are expected to change healthcare delivery in a number of different methods Findings, results or prescription which is not requiring face-to-face contact (such as prescription repeat) or important follow-up data of the patients can be collected remotely (such as blood glucose level measurements) are easily handled by telemedicine. For example:

• **ePSS:** The Electronic Preventive Services Selector (ePSS) is an application designed to help primary care clinicians identify the screening, counselling, and preventive medication services that are appropriate for their patients. The ePSS application is based on the current recommendations of the U.S. Preventive Services Task Force and can be searched by specific patient characteristics, such as age, sex, and selected behavioural risk factors.

• **Epocrates:** More than 50 evidence-based, patient-specific guidelines from national speciality societies which are condensed for the moments of care are available.

• **DRG:** It provides healthcare organizations and medical professionals with the data and guidance they need to bring potent, efficient therapies to patients around the world.

• In Turkey, **eNabiz (e-Pulse)** is a digital infrastructure that kept all data relating to patients within the health system through the application. Patients can share their data with healthcare personnel according to their level of authority. In this way, patients do not need to carry radiological images, prescriptions and laboratory results with them at every control visit.

• Intermountain Healthcare, USA, is a remote consultation system developed to assist in patient assessment and reduces the need for patients to obtain work permits when they need to get expert advice on simple issues.

• **CellScope Oto;** As mentioned above tympanic membrane image can be distantly shared with the help of CellScope Oto via smartphone by custom applications. Its clinical effectiveness is approved for otitis media.

• **MediGo**, Germany, introduced an app which facilitators can request a specialist second opinion. The application connects specialised doctors with medical tourism facilitator agents. A facilitator can send a question about the patient's request or clinical conditions; the application then directs questions to appropriate specialists or hospitals, who will review the patient's records and provide guidance.

• **Beyond Verbal** is an innovative voice-enabled AI solution for creating proprietary vocal biomarkers for individualized healthcare screening and continuous remote monitoring of health and emotions. It works on Vocal Biomarkers. Vocal Biomarkers can be gathered by free-form speech analysis, which provides non-intrusive, continuous and scalable information about patients' health.

• **mPower, Rochester University;** Since its launch in 2015, the mPower application by Rochester University has enrolled over ten thousand entrants, making it the largest Parkinson's study in history. The application helps researchers for understanding Parkinson's disease deeply by using the gyroscope and other iPhone features to measure dexterity, balance, gait, and memory. With the help of mPower app, researchers have obtained greater insight into the factors that causing symptoms better or worse, such as sleep, exercise, and mood.

• **EpiWatch, Johns Hopkins University;** With the help of Apple Watch, researchers planned a study to predict seizures before they happen. Since its launch, the EpiWatch application has enabled patients and practitioners to accurately track the onset and duration of seizures in real time, to create a correlation between seizures' episode history and medication. Patients sensing an impending seizure start the application by tapping Apple Watch. After starting the application, the accelerometer and heart rate sensors are triggered, and an alert is automatically sent to a designated family member or caregiver.

• **Autism & Beyond, Duke University, University of Cape Town;** Research has shown that early treatment of developmental problems can lead to higher IQs and better social skills. The Autism & Beyond application utilizes the front HD camera of iPhone, along with innovative facial recognition algorithms, to analyze emotional reactions to videos in children as young as 18 months. With the help of the app, children can be screened without having to see a specialist personally, allowing for earlier diagnosis and treatment.

• **DeepMind;** It is the London-based and Alphabet Inc. owned AI company that works on developing a medical product that will help doctors to detect sight-threatening circumstances from a common type of eye scan. It is a trained AI software to detect signs of eye disease better than physicians, according to study partners in the research, (Moorfields Eye Hospital and the University College London Institute of Ophthalmology).

New digital technology promises cost efficiency and better patient experience in the near term, but the adaptation of new technologies is slower than expected. Cost of new technology, fears for data-security, difficulties in educating the patients and staff, and resistance to change in healthcare practices are the main reasons for digital technology integration problems.

Patient involvement in healthcare

Technological transformation in health care has enabled patients to become stakeholders in health care. Individuals have taken responsibility for their health even before the disease situation has emerged, and they started to use AppleWatch, Samsung Watch and similar wearable technology. In addition, an increasing number of online health information sites and health-themed applications indicate that people are approaching the issue of healthy living positively. To manage these new trends, hospitals and governments are offering digital solutions to increase patients' involvement in, and visibility into, their care. In addition, a significant portion of health-related websites and mobile applications are now being prepared by major health care organizations and governments to avoid confusion as the value and importance of evidence-based health information is understood. Mobile health (mHealth) is a common term for the use of wireless technologies in healthcare. mHealth is a popular option in areas where there are a large population and widespread wireless device use. For people, a major benefit of mHealth is its convenience. Wearables and other mobile technologies allow individuals to ceaselessly track and manage specific health data. There are also a plethora of apps to choose from: There are almost 350,000 mHealth applications obtainable from app stores, according to research2guidance.

As before mentioned, in Turkey, a nationwide service, "e-Nabiz (e-Pulse)", allows people to schedule and cancel appointments online or mobile, view their EMRs, keep track prescriptions, and get support online. Similarly, in Sweden, a nationwide healthcare service, "1177 Vårdguiden", additionally to e-Nabiz abilities, it can also offer prescription renewal and treatment support.

Harnessing patient-generated data

Enlarged, spread and circulated data sets that include genetic, lifestyle, and physiological data can improve the sensitivity and specificity of medical diagnoses and treatment. Healthcare providers including governments are investing to collect more data across the population, precise risk factors causing disease, and specify biomarkers for an effective treatment. Furthermore, these kinds of data will also open a route for personalised treatment which offers reducing overall healthcare cost.

Today's healthcare world, most of the treatment decisions are based on guidelines and evidence of clinical trials or metadata. Many healthcare providers have started to use genetic tests for personalised treatment. For instance, The Dana-Farber/Harvard Cancer Center DNA Resource Core is a centralized laboratory that provides Sanger DNA sequencing and plasmid services to researchers in their community and around the world. They use DNA sequencing in leukaemia and lung cancer patients to decide personalised or definite targeted therapies. DNA sequencing not only for human, but it also gives great opportunity to specify microorganism and to find specific treatment options for microorganism.

Final Words

Increasing the training of medical professionals during their educational period on how to use new and existing technology is expanding and improving worldwide. The advancement and innovation of medical technologies have forced Australia to increase medical school numbers. In many countries, bold steps are being taken to develop medical technology infrastructure capacities and capabilities in order to follow and manage the rapidly developing innovations in health care. Advances in healthcare are not all in operating theatres laboratories. Digital technologies together with AI, automaton and robotics also changed the application and distribution of healthcare information. Thus, the roles of all healthcare professionals "from physicians to nurses" have widened and a new career route opened for all in relation in informatics and digitals.

Whether technological inventions and advancements are accepted as a threat or an opportunity to providing better care will depend upon "attitudes to technology and levels of tolerance" of physicians with alongside the health literacy level of the people. Above all, the effectiveness and accuracy of existing technology will provide an encouraging contribution to future innovative development. People may find diagnostic digital technology applications attractive for many reasons, such as user-friendliness, the ease of access and cost-effectiveness. In the near future, individuals will look for technologic solutions to their pathological conditions and expect the physicians to keep up with technological developments.

The physicians should advocate preventive medicine and should help to software developer for creating better digital solutions for detection and follow up of diseases so the software may direct patients towards appropriate medical care. The doctors should have taken advantage of the sophisticated diagnostic technologic capability of applications where possible.

References

1. Abbott L.M., Smith S.D.; Smartphone apps for skin cancer diagnosis: Implications for patients and practitioners; Australasian Journal of Dermatology (2018) 59, 168–170 doi: 10.1111/ajd.12758

2. Bold Business; Preparing Healthcare Workforce Technological Advancements; https://www.boldbusiness.com/health/preparing-healthcare-workforce-technological-advancements/ Accessed on 14 June 2019

3. BTOES Insights Official; Reducing The Utilization Of Continuous Observations For Safety Precautions; April 2017; http://insights.btoes.com/poster-presentation/winning-study-reducing-the-utilization-of-continuous-observations-for-safety-precautions Accessed on 11 June 2019

4. Camm J., Klein H., Nisam S., The cost of implantable defibrillators: perceptions and reality, European Heart Journal, Volume 28, Issue 4, February 2007, Pages 392–397, https://doi.org/10.1093/eurheartj/ehl166

5. Charmsaz, S., Prencipe, M., Kiely, M., Pidgeon, G. P., & Collins, D. M. (2018). Innovative Technologies Changing Cancer Treatment. Cancers, 10(6), 208. doi:10.3390/cancers10060208

6. Dash P., Henricson C., Kumar P., Stern N.; The hospital is dead, long live the hospital!; Mc Kinsey & Company, May 2019; 2-18

7. Degala S., (2018); Five innovation trends that will impact the healthcare industry in 2018 https://medcitynews.com/2018/12/five-innovation-trends-that-will-impact-the-healthcare-industry-in-2019/?rf=1 Accessed on 11 June 2019

8. Esteva A., Kuprel B., Novoa R.A., Ko J., Swetter S.M., Blau H.M., Thrun S., (2017); Dermatologist-level classification of skin cancer with deep neural networks; Nature volume542, pages115–118

9. Global Future of Work Center of Excellence (2016). Future of Work Disruptions Index. Deloitte UK. https://www2.deloitte.com/content/ dam/ Deloitte/ca/Documents/human-capital/ca-EN-HC-The-Intelligence-Revolution-FINAL-AODA.pdf.

10. Gombolay, M., Yang, X. J., Hayes, B., Seo, N., Liu, Z., Wadhwania, S., Yu T., Shah N., Golen T., Shah, J. (2018). Robotic assistance in the coordination of patient care. The International Journal of Robotics Research, 37(10), 1300–1316. https://doi.org/10.1177/0278364918778344

11. Healthcare Weekly Staff; 5 Innovations That Will Change the Treatment of Heart Disease; July 2018 https://healthcareweekly.com/five-innovations-in-heart-disease-treatment/

12. Heron M.; Deaths: Leading Causes for 2017, (2019); National Vital Statistics Reports, Vol. 68, No. 6, June 24, 2019

13. Hildreth C.; Cost Of Stem Cell Therapy And Why It's So Expensive (November 21, 2018) https://bioinformant.com/cost-of-stem-cell-therapy/ Accessed on 13 June 2019

14. Johnston K.; Hey robot, is that report ready? https://www.bostonglobe.com/business/2018/11/04/hey-robot-that-report-ready/LrGEKOLaBJB50MA8tzTXbP/story.html Accessed on 16 June 2019

15. Kahn J., Google's DeepMind To Create Product to Spot Eye Disease (August

2018); https://www.bloomberg.com/news/articles/2018-08-13/google-s-deepmind-to-create-product-to-spot-sight-threatening-disease Accessed on 13 June 2019

16. Larsen G., Hallstrom A., McAnulty J., Pinski S., Olarte A., Sullivan S., Brodsky M., Powell J., Marchant C., Jennings C., Akiyama T., the AVID Investigators Cost-effectiveness of the implantable cardioverter-defibrillator versus antiarrhythmic drugs in survivors of serious ventricular tachyarrhythmias: results of the Antiarrhythmics Versus Implantable Defibrillators (AVID) economic analysis substudy Circulation 2002; 105; 2049-2057

17. Manyika J, Sneader K. Automation and the future of work: Ten things to solve for. McKinsey Global Institute. June 2018.

18. Molteni M. If you look at X-rays or moles for a living, AI is coming for your job (2017); Wired, Available from URL: https://www.wired.com/2017/01/look-x-rays-moles-living-ai-coming-job/ (Accessed 20 June 2019.)

19. Rappaport, K. M., McCracken, C. C., Beniflah, J., Little, W. K., Fletcher, D. A., Lam, W. A., & Shane, A. L. (2016). Assessment of a Smartphone Otoscope Device for the Diagnosis and Management of Otitis Media. Clinical Pediatrics, 55(9), 800–810. https://doi.org/10.1177/0009922815593909

20. Roche E.T., Markus A. Horvath M.A., Wamala I., Alazmani A., Song S.E., Whyte W., Zurab Machaidze Z., Payne C.J., Weaver J.C., Fishbein G., Kuebler J., Vasilyev N.W., Mooney D.J., Pigula F.A., Walsh C.J.; Soft robotic sleeve supports heart function (2017); Science Translational Medicine; Vol. 9, Issue 373, eaaf3925 DOI: 10.1126/scitranslmed.aaf3925

21. Rouse M., (2018); mHealth (mobile health) https://searchhealthit.techtarget.com/definition/mHealth Accessed on 11 June 2019

22. Sahni N et al. The Productivity Imperative for Healthcare Delivery in the United States. McKinsey report. February 2019.

23. Sahyouni R, Moshtaghi O, Rajaii R. et al. Evaluation of an iPhone Otoscope in a Neurotrauma Clinic and as an Adjunct to Neurosurgical Education. Neurosurg. 2016, 2:1.

24. Schwartz J., Jennifer Radin J., Cooney J., Medlock M., Hays D., Sklar D.; Deloitte; The future is here, 2018 Deloitte Development LLC

25. Taylor K., 12 medical technology innovations likely to transform health care in 2017 (2017), https://blogs.deloitte.com/centerforhealthsolutions/12-medical-technology-innovations-likely-transform-health-care-2017/

26. Thomas S., Meet the Health Care Workforce of the Future; (2018); https://deloitte.wsj.com/cfo/2018/05/01/meet-the-health-care-workforce-of-the-future/ (Accessed 20 June 2019.)

27. Thorpe K.E., Florence C.S., Howard D.H., and Peter Joski "The Rising Prevalence of Treated Disease: Effects on Private Health Insurance Spending," Health Affairs, 27 June 2005 content.healthaffairs.org/cgi/content/abstract/hlthaff.w5.317 (25 August 2005).

28. Toussaint J.S., Berry L.L.; The Promise of Lean in Health Care; Mayo Clin. Proc. January 2013;88(1):74-82 http://dx.doi.org/10.1016/j.mayocp.2012.07.025

Chapter XIX

-

The Rise in Health Care Spending and Reform Proposals

by Dr. H. Omer TONTUS

The demand for efficient treatment technologies is growing every day, due to the need for cost-effective healthcare delivery. To increase the success rate of innovative treatment technologies, both governments and the private sector put more emphasis on the efficiency of the innovation process providing incentives, financial support and advisory services and facilities for testing and verification.

Reforms for decelerating the rise in healthcare expenditure and improving the value of care have greatly focused on the reimbursement systems. However, most of the rise in healthcare cost over the last decade is linked to lifestyle-related risk factors such as obesity and smoking. Increasing disease prevalence and recently developed treatments options charges for nearly 60% of the rise in expenditure. For effective reforms, policy-makers should focus on health promotion, preventive medicine, and the cost-effective use of healthcare. Answers for reducing health related expenditure growth is public health and preventive interventions.

Health insurance costs are steadily rising. Many researchers have been linked this permanent rise to the low out-of-pocket costs paid by consumers. The expenditure growth of healthcare has also been dependent to increased use of prescription drugs and over-used new costly medical innovations and treatments.

To fill a pool, it is necessary both to provide water flow to the pool and to prevent water leakage from the pool. Similarly, in order to reduce health expenditures, it is necessary to reduce the cost of medical care and to combat disease-causing conditions.

Efforts to reduce health system costs involve national confusing conflicts. In order to reduce health expenses, the efforts to promote healthy lifestyle preference which should be done first, are almost non-existent when compared with the works that promote tobacco and unhealthy nutrition.

However, almost 65% of the increase in healthcare spending is related to a rise in treated chronic diseases prevalence (e.g. diabetes) and innovations in medical treatment options. Habits such as unhealthy diet, lack of activity, tobacco usage and stress are the reason for about 50% of morbidity and mortality. Although the increase in health care demand has a significant impact on health-based expenditures, it is not correct to attribute increased health expenditures to patient-only reasons. There are multifactorial reasons behind the increase in health expenditures that can vary according to time and place.

Many countries' (such as Turkey and the USA) cost-control policy has focused too narrowly on demand-side interventions. There isn't any country where governments' plans to reduce health care costs by paying the least to service providers through reimbursement agencies were successful. In Turkey, for example, despite all the fragile balance in economic data of country and exchange rate fluctuations "package price list" of healthcare has never been changed significantly in favour of the healthcare providers about the last 10 years. However, in the same period, the minimum wage increased by approximately 383%. Consequently, personnel expenditures, which is the most important cost of health facilities, have increased significantly. While the cost of healthcare facilities increases, their income is kept under control by public policymakers. it seems that in the short term, the expenditure for the healthcare of governments may be reduced but in the long term, the price will be the plummeted patient satisfaction level which is resulted by the erosion of trust in government policies.

This chapter summarizes the components which are responsible for the increase in healthcare expenditure. As the works of literature indicate, most of the increase has been driven by a leap in treated diseases' prevalence which pushed by a rise in factors such as obesity and limited daily activity and by innovations in the treatment of chronic diseases. The papers indicate a series of reforms that are designed to address the factors responsible for the increase in expenditure.

The Rise In Healthcare Spendings

First of all, let's give a simple example of our daily life. If you buy 1 apple every day and pay $1 for each apple, you will spend $ 365 a year. If the number of apples you receive per day increases, for example, if you buy 2 apples, you will have to pay more in total, even if the apple price decreases by 25%. Similarly, the growth in healthcare spending is simply related to the growth in the number of medical conditions treated. Other reasons for the increase in health care expenditures is the new but expensive types of treatment that have emerged with the changing treatment options, and the treatment of previously untreated diseases. Consequently, both the increase in the number of patients (due to population growth and ageing) and the increase in cost per treatment significantly increase the total expenditure related to health services.

If we evaluate the Table 5 at this point, the number of cases treated for 20 different diseases (per 100.000) and per-case treatment costs are seen from 1987 to 2002. The number of patients treated for 3 diseases decreased within 15 years (Newborn and maternity care, Infectious disease, Bronchitis). Similarly, cost per case treatment for 3 diseases was reduced (Mental disorders, Upper gastrointestinal, Cerebrovascular disease). However, there was no effect of decreasing health expenses due to the increase in cost per case treatment of these diseases with the decrease in treated prevalence. A total of $6,159,182 was spent for 22664 cases in 1987 per 100,000 people for these three disease groups. A total of $ 19,113,888 was spent on 20418 cases in 2002 for every 100,000 people for the same diseases. In other words, although treatment prevalence decreased by approximately 10%, treatment cost increased by 310%. When we examine the 3 diseases with a reduced cost per case treatment, we encounter a similar situation. As can be seen from the table, the cost of treatment per case related to 3 diseases decreased within 15 years (Mental disorders, Upper gastrointestinal, Cerebrovascular disease). However, the decrease in per-case treatment costs had no effect on decreasing health costs due to the increase in the prevalence of diseases. A total of $ 9.052.192 was spent on 7,408 cases in 1987 per 100,000 people for these three disease groups. A total of $ 17,727,736 was spent on 18,371 cases in 2002 for every 100,000 people for the same diseases. In other words, although the cost per case was reduced, the total cost increased by 196% due to the increase in the number of cases.

For these 20 diseases in per 100,000 people, 69 million dollars were spent in 1987 and 134.4 million dollars were spent in 2002. Therefore, it is seen that health expenditures for these diseases have increased approximately twice in 15 years. But, when we connect with the total US population in the same years, we see that in 1987, 167.4 billion dollars were spent on these diseases and in 2002, 395.5 billion dollars were spent. Therefore, health expenditures for these diseases have increased by 2.36 times by not only the effect of population increase also effect of cost per treatments and prevalence.

Medical condition	Case Number per 100000		Cost per treatment		Spending for per 100000		Total cost change
	1987	2002	1987	2002	1987	2002	
Newborn and maternity care	3.406	2.940	773	3.950	2.632.838	11.613.000	441%
Cancer	2.710	3.666	3.081	3.999	8.349.510	14.660.334	176%
Pulmonary conditions	9.294	17.699	507	639	4.712.058	11.309.661	240%
Arthritis	4.573	7.640	701	1.282	3.205.673	9.794.480	306%
Mental disorders	4.658	10.984	1.242	972	5.785.236	10.676.448	185%
Hyperlipidemia	1.383	7.427	278	618	384.474	4.589.886	1194%
Hypertension	9.372	11.988	456	664	4.273.632	7.960.032	186%
Lupus	4.177	6.535	470	868	1.963.190	5.672.380	289%
Back problems	4.581	8.144	1.457	1.202	6.674.517	9.789.088	147%
Upper gastrointestinal	2.622	7.042	854	769	2.239.188	5.415.298	242%
Diabetes	2.420	3.972	1.293	1.551	3.129.060	6.160.572	197%
Kidney problems	662	1.318	3.918	4.101	2.593.716	5.405.118	208%
Infectious disease	5.858	5.793	268	726	1.569.944	4.205.718	268%
Heart disease	4.610	5.002	2.734	2.753	12.603.740	13.770.506	109%
Skin disorders	6.695	9.144	344	471	2.303.080	4.306.824	187%
Bronchitis	13.400	11.685	146	282	1.956.400	3.295.170	168%
Endocrine disorders	6.402	7.906	389	467	2.490.378	3.692.102	148%
Other gastrointestinal diseases	1.280	2.461	664	848	849.920	2.086.928	246%
Bone disorders	620	2.030	555	700	344.100	1.421.000	413%
Cerebrovascular disease	132	345	7.812	4.742	1.031.184	1.635.990	159%
Total spending for per 100000					69.091.838	137.460.535	199%
Population					242.300.000	287.600.000	119%
Total expenditure projected to the population					167.409.523.474	395.336.498.660	236%

Table 5 - Change in treated disease prevalence and its impact on private insurance spending

Adopted from Thorpe K.E. et al content.healthaffairs.org/cgi/content/abstract/hlthaff.w5.317

It is natural that as the population increases and gets older, more cases will be treated and innovative treatment solutions will have the extra cost. However, with the help of preventive medicine, it is possible to avoid serious complications by protecting individuals from certain clinical situations. For example, obesity and tobacco use cause many different diseases and clinical symptoms and increase the risk of complications of diseases. Therefore, campaigns to provide individuals with a healthy life culture to combat these two issues will contribute to the reduction of health care costs. Obesity seems important enough to be an independent title for future health expenditures. Many studies have shown a direct relationship between obesity and diseases such as diabetes, back pain, some cardiovascular diseases, hyperlipidemia, and hypertension. Thus, the increase in the rate of obesity increases not only the costs associated with the treatment of obese patients but also the costs of comorbid or obesity-related disease treatments.

Table 6 shows the changes from 2000 to 2012, it is seen that both the number of cases treated and the cost of treatment per case have increased over the years. It can be said that the cost increase per case has slowed down in the last 4 years (2008-2012).

When we look at the table by assuming that there are 100 cases in 2000 by as a base and that we spend $100 for each case, it is seen that the number of cases in 2012 reached to 125 and that the expenditure per case was reached $167. In this case, in 2000, $ 10,000 was paid for 100 cases and in 2012, $ 20901 paid for 125 cases. As it is seen from the table that the population growth rate is 11.23% in the same period, it will be seen that the increase in the number of cases is more than twice the population growth rate. This indicates an increase in health expenditures of approximately 109%.

According to the World Bank data, the US GDP per capita for the year 2000 was $36334,909 and in 2012 it was $51603,497. The GDP growth rate was 42.02%. In short, for the US, the increase in health expenditures is higher than the population growth rate and per capita GDP growth. It is clear that health spending growth has outpaced growth of the U.S. economy.

Year	Change on Cost per case	Change on Number of treated cases	Cumulative change on cost per case	Cumulative change on number of treated case	Population (in million)
2000	Base	Base	100,00	100,00	282,16
2001	8,5%	1,1%	108,50	101,10	284,97
2002	5,6%	3,5%	114,58	104,64	287,63
2003	6,9%	0,5%	122,48	105,16	290,11
2004	6,0%	1,5%	129,83	106,74	292,81
2005	3,6%	2,7%	134,50	109,62	295,52
2006	3,7%	2,8%	139,48	112,69	298,38
2007	4,3%	1,7%	145,48	114,61	301,23
2008	2,4%	2,4%	148,97	117,36	304,09
2009	3,9%	1,2%	154,78	118,77	306,77
2010	3,4%	0,5%	160,04	119,36	309,33
2011	2,3%	2,4%	163,72	122,22	311,58
2012	2,1%	2,3%	167,16	125,03	313,87

Table 6 - Percent change from previous year for price indexes and real expenditures on medical services by disease, 2001 - 2012

Lifestyle Choice and effects on healthcare

Changes in lifestyle could prevent many of the chronic illnesses which are rising up healthcare expenditures, also with improving health it could reduce the need for costly treatments. In 2016, the US healthcare spending for chronic diseases such as heart disease, cancer, diabetes, and Alzheimer's disease amounted to $1.1 trillion. When lost economic productivity is added, the economic impact of chronic diseases goes up to $3.7 trillion. This is almost 20% of the US GDP. In terms of risk factors, being overweight or obese accounts for $ 1.7 trillion or 47% of the total cost. About 8.7% of US health care spending is for smoking; 60% of this is paid by public resources. Health problems resulting from excessive drinking cost over $ 27 billion in 2010. These diseases, which increase rapidly due to the choice of lifestyle, put a serious burden on the whole health system, especially the hospitals, and even on the national economies. The most rapid way for lowering chronic disease-related costs, or at least to slow the rising, is to reduce the number of people who are with excess weight, smokes, or drinks too much alcohol. For example, according to 2016 data, 40% of American adults are classified as obese, while 33% are defined as overweight.

The obesity prevalence in the U.S. has increased consistently from 3.4% of adults in 1962 to 39.8% in 2016, the year of the most recent CDC data. In 2016, 180.5 million people ages 2 and over were either obese or overweight, which is equivalent to more than 60%

of the total population. In 2016, chronic diseases driven by obesity and overweight cost almost $481 billion in direct healthcare expenses in the U.S., with an additional $1.24 trillion in indirect expenses due to lost economic productivity. The total cost of chronic diseases due to obesity and overweight was equivalent to 9.3% of the U.S. GDP, in 2016.

Epidemiological and clinical researches have shown a potent relationship between obesity and chronic diseases such as heart disease, kidney disease, type 2 diabetes and arthritis. Therefore, it is expected that such a high percentage of obese and overweight individuals will have a negative impact on the American economy due to increased health expenditures.

Financial incentives for weight loss, exercise and smoking cessation can be provided, as well as public awareness and health education campaigns promoting a healthy lifestyle. Infrastructure improvements can encourage more people to walk, jog and bike. In addition, studies can be conducted to reduce the salt, fat, sugar and other unhealthy additives in the products of food companies. The North Karelia Project is an example of a very successful campaign for such planning. The project, which has been going on for more than twenty years, has been educated on the dangers of healthier eating, more exercise and the use of tobacco products. As a result, in the early 1970s in Finland, North Karelia had the highest rate of heart attacks in the world, while the North Karelia project led to a 63% reduction in coronary heart disease deaths for men aged 30 to 64 years.

Obesity and overweight as a risk factor are by far the greatest contributor to chronic diseases which are linked to 75% of osteoarthritis cases, 64% of Type 2 diabetes cases, 73% of kidney disease cases. Obesity and the burden of chronic diseases have reached record economic heights, and new records continue to be broken every year in a row. Without any doubt, more effective weight-control strategies could reduce both the health and economic burdens of chronic diseases. Many studies have shown that prevention is much cheaper than treatment, but it is difficult to change health-related behaviours.

Effects of changed clinical limits for treatment

Changes in clinical limits for treatment also have resulted in more patients' being treated for even asymptomatic conditions. This reflects especially the preventive treatment protocol for individuals with hypercholesterolemia, high blood pressure and DM, which are cardiac disease risk factors. Cut-off limits have changed many times within the last half a century. When I was a young family medicine practitioner in the late '80s prescription limit for blood pressure was 160/95 mmHg (systolic/diastolic) which is changed to 140/90 in the early 2000s. This threshold limit change led to the prescription for millions of additional patients with the cost to the healthcare system. Similar was the case for blood cholesterol level and for heart rate. As the relationship between hypertension and renal diseases leading to renal failure and cerebrovascular diseases is better-understood, and new recommendations for treatment plans have started to be made at lower blood pressure limits in terms of preventive medicine.

Approximately 23 million adults are estimated to have high-normal blood pressure readings of 130–139/85–89 mm Hg. Similar threshold change has recommended in lipidemia control, the level for treatment has dropped from 240 down to 200 for total cholesterol levels. 13 Another important threshold is announced for diabetes for preventive medicine, treatment level for fasting glucose levels declined from 110 to 100. More than 10 millions of Americans now are "pre-diabetic" and they need prescriptions and insurance coverage.

As a result of these varying thresholds, the number of treated adults increased sharply. The question is whether further aggressive treatment and control will result in improved cardiovascular outcomes and whether additional expenditure can lead to even greater improvements in health outcomes. Some evaluations suggest that increased use of antihypertensive drugs and statin drugs is associated with the desired reductions among adults in recent years. But we will never really know how much these reductions are protecting people from possible cardiac disease. Therefore, it is not easy to make a realistic cost-effectiveness analysis. However, it is obvious that these changes create a significant cost burden that future health system managers need to solve.

Effect of Innovations to Treatment

Innovations in medical treatment have an important effect on the expanding of treated disease and individuals. The positive effects of medical innovations are indisputable. The struggle against infectious diseases such as tuberculosis, malaria, pneumonia, and typhoid fever was won. With the innovation of antibiotics, deaths from the infectious disease plummeted swiftly and were no longer common after the 60s. Thus, life expectancy increased as a result. These diseases were replaced by diabetes, heart diseases, stroke, mental illnesses, and cancers. Both the changes in the pharmacological field and the new options developed in the treatment protocols reflected as the increasing cost to health systems.

Latest innovations in medicine are revolutionizing medical practice. At the same time, characteristics of the diseases are changing and the proportion of the elderly in the population is increasing. As healthier individuals live longer, cumulative health expenditures increase due to illness and disability, as expected. There is a substantial risk in future healthcare spending due to the increasing elderly population, and it is unlikely a "magical touch" will be found to both for improving health and dramatically reducing medical expenditure. Therefore, there is a need to develop cost-effective innovative technologies. As in all sectors, it should be expected that every new invention will have a cost in the period until it becomes widespread. Medical innovative solutions can also be predicted to be costly at least during the first 5-10 years.

For example, a sharp increase in expenditure per newborn with low birth weight is directly related to innovative technologies aimed at improving survival rates. For this survival rate improvement, the number of newborn intensive care beds in the hospital was increased, more doctors were trained as neonatal-ICU specialists, new multi-parameter incubators were developed and new model ventilators were produced. These are all high-cost transactions. The allocation of more space for newborns in hospitals restricts the space to be used for other income generating activities. However, special training for both physicians and nurses to gain special expertise on neonatal-ICU results in less patient-physician interaction for them. This costly training creates a burden on the healthcare system and also removes this group of professionals from faster income generating medical activities. Newly developed molecules have a special place in health expenditures. For example, for the treatment of depression alone, the prescription of the psychotropic drug for patients (or people) increased from 45% in 1987 to about 80% in the early 2000s.

Heart diseases are the most common cause of death in the world for many years. According to the CDC report dated June 24, 2019, 22,99% of the deaths in the US in 2017 were caused by heart disease and 22,03% were caused by malignant neoplasm. Depending on the U.S. statistics one American dies of cardiovascular disease every 38 seconds, which costs the healthcare system more than $330 billion a year. Because of that, the medical device producer and/or pharmacy companies are working to find innovative solutions to heart diseases.

Implications For Health Care Reform Proposals

As defined above, most of the rise in healthcare expenditure can be based on the increase in obesity and new medical technologies. Much of the recent controversy about health care reform has been focused on demand-side reforms and individual-driven health plans. This approach is a populist approach that will not have any effect on keeping health expenditures under control or stopping the increase even if it is accepted individually. The so-called primary health care reforms, such as fewer contributions, right to further benefit, unlimited physician visits, will not be able to solve the rising cost problem of healthcare in the long term.

For example, in Turkey in the early 2000s made health care reform with the satisfaction of the public health services has increased over a decade. The goal of meeting the demand that was at the center of the reform resulted in the demand and consumption of health services that could not be met in 10 years. As a result, an even more costly solution was created for the unmet demand, thus increasing the number of hospitals. In 2017, the total number of applications to hospitals was 464.8 million. In the same year, there were approximately 90,200 doctors in all units and 5153 patients applied per physician. The number of doctoral visits per person increased from 3.2 in 2002 to 8.2 in 2011 with a steady increase, and this shows that policy development focused on meeting the demand cannot be a solution. For the planning of healthcare reform, Turkey's " Program of Transformation in Health" is a good example with "do's and don'ts" lessons as well. Healthcare is costly and increasing demand will have a devastating impact on public finances, even if the cost per case is reduced.

Surely, this is not to say that demand-side interventions should not be pursued; they should be. Instead, the analysis indicates that an extensive list of reforms, including public health and population-based interventions and more effective models for treating chronic diseases, should be at the core of reform efforts to slow healthcare expenditure growth.

Countries that focus on the fight against only tobacco use, which has more populist effects, have unfortunately put the fight against obesity in the second place. The most obvious example of this, sad to say, still given as Turkey. Although Turkey received several achievement awards from WHO in the field of the fight against tobacco, there was the unsatisfactory fight against obesity in the 2000s.

Additionally, more than 75% of healthcare expenditure is spent on patients with largely predictable healthcare needs and chronical diseases. Finally, the faster adoption of poorly structured and consumer-oriented populist reform plans by governments has done little to do with the increase in obesity, stress and other population risk factors that have led to an increase in the prevalence of disease over the past two decades. But populist healthcare transformation reform plans have resulted in disastrous cost for economies.

Subjects For Potential Reforms

The subjects that cause cost increases in health care provision and which should be considered by policymakers can be listed as follows:

1- As the cultural structure, level of knowledge and understanding change, people become interested in diseases that they did not care about before. Developments such as urbanization, better public transport, developed online hospital appointment systems and increased supply of services have led to the patients "more quickly and easily get serviced" have become the reason for the more hospital visit. The discomforts or symptoms (e.g. sub-febrile fever) that can be solved by traditional methods, day by day is causing more outpatient clinic admission.

2- While health services have become complex and comprehensive with rapid technological development and professional differentiation, the new rules and regulations of many countries have failed to keep up with this rapid change and despite the increasing workload, the service has been focused on physicians' workforce. Today, many jobs that do not require training and skills at the physician level are placed on the physicians' shoulder. Although, for 2019-2020 educational year 15050 positions opened for students for medical school enrolment in Turkey only 14000 positions opened for nursing school enrolment. This is an important finding that regulating bodies do not copy the healthcare sector's needs.

3- Management model changes, such as patient-oriented service understanding, empowerment of the patient in the system and participation in decision-making processes, constitute a process managed by the patient's perception, understanding and expectations, not "evidence-based" behaviours. In countries and regions where health literacy is low, this change results in more hospital visits by individuals.

4. In the past, when a diagnosis is made using limited diagnostic tools and the appropriate treatment is chosen, a wide variety of technological diagnostic methods are now used. The use of expensive diagnostic methods rather than simple and conventional techniques is preferred by both patients and physicians. This leads to both higher patient density and unnecessary health expenditure.

5. Campaigns related to disease prevention and early detection may raise suspicion about individuals to own health. Therefore, there should be harmony between the language used in the campaigns and the health-literacy of the target audience.

6- Regular monthly medical examinations and follow-up of pregnant women and babies should be performed in primary health care centers. Health centers should have the infrastructure to provide follow-up of these individuals. It is important that such follow-ups can be solved without the need for hospital visits. Otherwise, this group may cause unnecessary concentration and waiting list in hospitals.

7- Services such as health screening and check-up to recognize neglected and disregarded health problems can be used as a means of producing patients by private health institutions, unethically.

8- Emergency departments can be seen as easy and fast access areas by the patients after working hours and are therefore overused. This situation, which causes unnecessary concentration in emergency services, also carries the risk of preventing the providing of necessary health services to real emergency cases.

9- As the health service sector is transformed into a trade sector, methods are developed to maximize profit and patient demand is produced for the bigger cake and bigger slice. Health institutions encourage people to apply because they benefit from patients' visits.

In addition, the relationship between the number of patients and the income of health care workers causes doctors to encourage patients to visit repeatedly which ultimately increase health expenditures. The fact that social insurance services have been opened for private health care institutions has enabled them to mobilize their own dynamics in attracting peoples as patients.

10. Social insurance systems in some countries have made health care accessible in a financial sense and have eliminated the cost factor, which is the main obstacle to almost everyone accessing it. Due to the ease of access, it is also possible that patients consult many doctors for the same illness or same symptoms in search of alternative opinions.

11. With the increasing communication channels such as social media, publicity and advertisements announce service alternatives and patients tend to apply to different doctors. Increased communication channels are also promoting the spread of inaccurate exaggerated information about health which resulted in information pollution. This is resulting in the increased health service consumption and demand for care. Policy-makers must build regulations for information sharing on the disease and the treatment, all sharing must be based on evidence-based information.

12- An important feature of health services is that supply (such as sophisticated buildings, up-to-date technological infrastructures) itself creates demand. The increase in opportunities, preferences and guidance for healthcare service chain are increasing the demand for services.

Costs And Benefits Of New Medical Technologies

New healthcare policies and reforms probably will target high-cost and low-benefit medical technologies.

With expanded data capacity, the healthcare systems would benefit from examining the costs and benefits associated with new and existing health care technologies. This will provide a wide range of information to policymakers about safeness, usefulness, cost-effectiveness, and differences, of new drugs or new technologies.

For example, ALLHAT (Anti-hypertensive and Lipid-Lowering Treatment to Prevent Heart Attack Trial) researchers examined the primary effects of antihypertensive drugs among DM-type 2, on fatal coronary heart disease and nonfatal myocardial infarction. The randomized study found that the cheapest drugs (a diuretic) were as effective as new very expensive drugs (ACE inhibitors).

Developing financial incentives for physicians and patients to use cost-effective treatments when the clinical and economic evidence is clear should be a key policy priority. However, this issue requires a very sensitive evaluation. For example, establishing a rule for prescribing high-cost drugs only by the relevant specialist physician may prevent patients' access to the drug at the right time.

Impact Factors Od Health Spendings

It is clear that no reform that does not foresee the fight against obesity, tobacco use, and a sedentary lifestyle can be successful. Healthcare reforms around the fight against chronic disease care rather than around building new hospitals would be an important subject. This would allow patients and insurers to compare the cost of treatment as well as the extent to which clinically appropriate medical care is provided. "Value"-focused policies based reforms highly probably can encourage the use of cost-effective health care.

As shown in Graphic 7, population increase, ageing, obesity and tobacco use have an effect on increasing the number of patients and health promotion studies have an effect on decreasing the number of patients. The increasing number of patients and the rise in the type of disease being treated have a direct impact on total healthcare expenditures. The medical tourism and health promotion activities as shown in the Graphic 7 have a decreasing effect on healthcare expenditures. The introduction of new drugs and the use of new technologies in health care have both cost-increasing and reducing effects. New drugs often appear to have high drug prices due to their right to development. However, it can be predicted that it will decrease the cost by increasing treatment success in the medium term. The same applies to technological innovations.

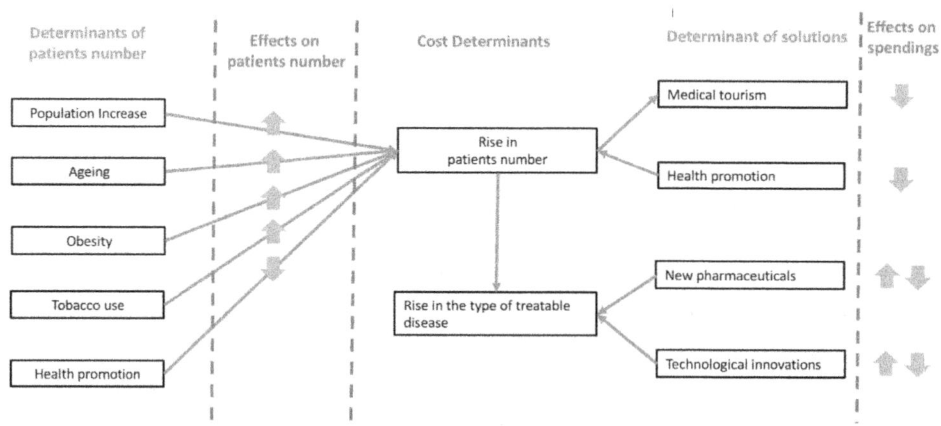

Graphic 7 - Factors of Health Spending

New Delivery Models And Impact On Healthcare

New healthcare service models for growing chronic care demands are bringing to the table by policymakers and experts. AI, Digital technologies and robotics will have key roles to play. Advancements in precise detection and diagnoses of the disease will go far to minimise the cost of treating chronic conditions. Advances in the definitive diagnosis of the diseases will be important to minimize the cost of treatment of chronic conditions. Genome sequencing and molecular diagnostics have enabled physicians to better understand the characteristics of diseases and develop sensitive personalized treatments.

Every new drug, every new device, every new software or application that enters the health sector is expanding and reshaping the healthcare system. The public sector, which is the main actor in the sector, naturally gives priority and more importance to preventive health solutions and patient-centred care. By the strong standing of public institutions, the demands of governments and the regulations put into practice, national or international companies are working on alternative answers to bring innovative solutions to chronic disease prevention and management difficulties. This opens the door to industries such as retail, telecommunications, technology, health tourism and well-being that are strengthened by their relationship with the health sector.

Due to the intense pressures on health systems, increasing costs, ageing society and the healthcare workforce shortage, international cooperation becomes necessary. As a matter of fact, governments are seeking and introducing solutions to balance rising financial burdens and facilitate access to health services. For example, the European Union (EU) provides promising solutions for a jointly applicable health system alliance. With the issued directive acts, a citizen of an EU country could be treated in another EU country and reimbursement institutions were able to pay for cross-border services. Similar collaborations take place on the basis of cost and service efficiency as cross-border health services within the scope of health tourism and this rapidly developing new solution can be expected to cover all countries.

The new healthcare delivery models are emerging as the concept of borders is blurred by worldwide, and access to medical institutions which having sophisticated technological infrastructures are getting more easy day by day. Economically and geopolitically powerful countries forces work to create a more dynamic and competitive marketplace. Therefore, adaptive operating models and accredited institutions can show flexibility on pricing and funding. One of the major challenges facing healthcare delivery systems is the likelihood that an operating system will invade healthcare delivery, as is the case with five-star hotels around the world. Many hotels contribute a very small portion of their income to the economy of the country in which they located. Similarly, a problem is likely to occur in the provision of health care in the medium term. This can clearly be seen as an exploit model of the 21st-century.

Final Words

Chronic diseases and conditions alongside with ageing population are on the rise globally. Costly chronic disease care needs are growing and applying considerable weight for healthcare systems. Ageing population and changes in lifestyle attitudes also are causing growth in expensive long-term health problems.

Especially in developing countries, the middle class is expanding; and with urbanisation growing, people are adopting more sedentary life habits, which causes a rise in obesity rates and chronic diseases such as diabetes. As stated by the WHO, chronic disease prevalence is expected to rise, and increased demand for healthcare systems due to chronic diseases has become a major concern and more will.

Another rising healthcare problem is global pandemic diseases. The very last pandemics have clearly demonstrated the speed of infections spread across the globe. For fighting with infectious diseases such as Ebola, SARS, and MERS, there is a need for internationally coordinated healthcare activities. Healthcare organisations especially governmental bodies all around the world need to be ready to work together as quickly as when pandemics occur.

Governments responsibilities are appraisals of technological advancements in healthcare, including assessments of health promotion programs. These appraisals should examine the cost increments and health benefits associated with drugs, medical instruments, diagnostic methods, and surgical interventions as well as health promotion activities. Thus, the policies and reforms process must include both medical and population interventions designed to improve health. For these reasons, planned policies and reforms should be designed to improve health, and include interventions and solutions for health professionals, the community and reimbursement agencies.

In order for new reforms or new policies to be effective, they must include both public and private sector interests. As stated before, governments are responsible for examining scientific evidence concerning the comparative clinical effectiveness, outcomes, and appropriateness of care.

Even if the studies to reduce the prevalence of common diseases specific to target audiences are not considered as a populist approach, it is a strategy with great potential benefits. For this reason, while developing cost-effective policies in health systems of the future; the implementation of AI, the use of digital technologies, robotic solutions, and the need to integrating health promotion solutions into healthcare is very important.

References:

1. Aydin S., Hekime başvuru sayısının artış hikâyesi (2015); Sağlik Dusuncesi ve Tip Kulturu Dergisi, 2015; 35; 6-13
2. CaringForDiabetes.com , "Screening and Diagnosis of Prediabetes and Metabolic Syndrome" www.caringfordiabetes.com/ScreeningandDiagnosis/Prediabetes/prediabetes.cfm (7 October 2005).
3. Cox C., Kaiser Family Foundation; How much does the U.S. spend to treat different diseases? (2017); https://www.healthsystemtracker.org/chart-collection/much-u-s-spend-treat-different-diseases/#item-cost-per-case-grown-faster-number-treated-cases-years-since-2001 Accessed 13 June 2019
4. Cutler D., Your Money or Your Life: Strong Medicine for America's Health Care System (New York: Oxford University Press, 2004). Google Scholar
5. Gregg E.W. et al., "Secular Trends in Cardiovascular Disease Risk Factors According to Body Mass Index in U.S. Adults," Journal of the American Medical

Association 293 , no. 15 (2005): 1868 –1874. Crossref, Medline , Google Scholar
6. Healthcare Weekly Staff; 5 Innovations That Will Change the Treatment of Heart Disease; July 2018 https://healthcareweekly.com/five-innovations-in-heart-disease-treatment/ Accessed 13 June 019
7. Henry J. Kaiser Family Foundation, Employer Health Benefits: 2004 Annual Survey, September 2004,www.kff.org/insurance/7148/index.cfm (26 August 2005). Google Scholar
8. Herrick D.M., Consumer Driven Health Care: The Changing Role of the Patient, NCPA Policy Heron M.; Deaths: Leading Causes for 2017, (2019); National Vital Statistics Reports, Vol. 68, No. 6, June 24, 2019
9. McGinnis J.M., Foege W.H., "Actual Causes of Death in the United States," Journal of the American Medical Association 270 , no. 18 (1993): 2207 –2212. Crossref, Medline See also M. Wolz et al., "Statement from the National High Blood Pressure Education Program: Prevalence of Hypertension," American Journal of Hypertension13 , no. 1, Part 1 (2000): 103 –104. Crossref, Medline , Google Scholar
10. McGinnis J.M., Williams-Russo P., Knickman J.R.,, "The Case for More Active Policy Attention to Health Promotion," Health Affairs 21 , no. 2 (2002): 78 –93. Medline , Google Scholar
11. Olfson M. et al., "National Trends in the Outpatient Treatment of Depression," Journal of the American Medical Association 287 , no. 2 (2002): 203 –209. Crossref , Google Scholar
12. PwC Global, Chronic diseases and conditions are on the rise; https://www.pwc.com/gx/en/industries/healthcare/emerging-trends-pwc-healthcare/chronic-diseases.html
13. Thorpe K.E., Florence C.S., Howard D.H., and Peter Joski "The Rising Prevalence of Treated Disease: Effects on Private Health Insurance Spending," Health Affairs, 27 June 2005 content.healthaffairs.org/cgi/content/abstract/hlthaff.w5.317 (25 August 2005).
14. Waters H., Graf M., Chronic diseases are taxing our health care system and our economy (2018); https://www.statnews.com/2018/05/31/chronic-diseases-taxing-health-care-economy/ Accessed 13 June 2019
15. Waters H., Graf M., America's Obesity Crisis, The Health And Economic Costs Of Excess Weight (2018) https://www.milkeninstitute.org/sites/default/files/reports-pdf/Mi-Americas-Obesity-Crisis-WEB.pdf October 2018
16. Whelton P.K. et al., "Clinical Outcomes in Antihypertensive Treatment of Type 2 Diabetes, Impaired Fasting Glucose Concentration, and Normoglycemia," Archives of Internal Medicine 165 , no. 12 (2005): 1401 –1409. Crossref, Medline ,

Chapter XX

-

An Important Solution for Future of Healthcare Delivery: Globalisation & Medical tourism

by Dr. H. Omer TONTUS

This chapter provides an outline of the current literature and facts about medical tourism and its possible impact on healthcare delivery in the future. Medical tourism plays a significant role in shaping the future of medical care worldwide, due to the growth of technology, economy, and other global relations. In accordance with tourism segment classification depending on journey reasons recommended by World Tourism Organization, one of the main groups is for "medical treatment/health". Being part of healthcare tourism, medical tourism is often called medical travel because it includes the act of travelling to different countries for medical reasons.

As a burgeoning industry globally, medical tourism can be accepted as an improvement of the healthcare system, which provides quality medical care to individuals seeking treatment. Carrera and Bridges defined healthcare tourism as pre-organized travel out of the local environment for the maintenance, enhancement or restoration of well-being in mind and body. Expansion in medical tourism has been facilitated by the rise of the internet, intercountry healthcare contracts, faster/cheaper travel opportunities, and the emergence of healthcare intermediaries or medical tourism facilitators between international patients and hospital networks. Some researcher such as Connell examined medical tourism-related studies in the literature to evaluate the extent, the longevity, the growth, and the trend of the sector, indicating that MT is likely to expand even faster in the near future. Connell also reported that most of the medical travels are short distance and diasporic, despite being part of an increasingly global sector. Quality and availability of care are key drivers of medical tourism behaviour, alongside economic and cultural factors.

Medical tourism is the product of "globalization in healthcare" and neoliberal policies. It is resulting from factors such as the persistent search for lower costs, higher quality care and shorter waiting lists. Medical travellers are individuals who travel internationally for non-emergency medical treatments such as organ transplants, oncological therapies, stem cell treatments, reproductive medicine, cosmetic surgery, and dental care. High costs, lack of insurance, under-insured, need for treatment outside insurance coverage, long waiting-times, and domestically unavailable treatments are some of the causes to go abroad to seek healthcare services. The major drivers for MT's fast growth are fueled by the rising costs of medical treatment and fluctuations of the global economy. As a comparison, charges for common procedures such as a heart bypass can be 10:1 between the US and Thailand, or 4:1 between the United States and Turkey for knee replacement. These kinds of cost differences in medical treatment are pushing the patients to cross-border medical travel from the US.

At the 9th National Health Conference having taken place in Rostock, Germany in 2013, medical tourism was defined as a subdomain under the healthcare and tourism industry contributing to maintaining and recovering health in general and wellness in particular, using approved medical services. Medical travels are not only a journey in order to improve health, but it is an economic activity implying service trade, representing a merge of at least two economic sectors: tourism and medicine. Medical tourism generates direct foreign exchange income and contributes to the overall development of any economy. It also provides employment and business opportunities for residents. Moreover, it aids the growth of associated businesses such as pharmaceuticals, medical devices, and tourism. Governmental support for country branding with the general reputation and political stability of the host country are key factors for driving the medical tourism market. Medical tourism has led to a rise in state-of-the-art medical facilities in developing countries to attract foreign patients, resulting in fast growth of healthcare infrastructure.

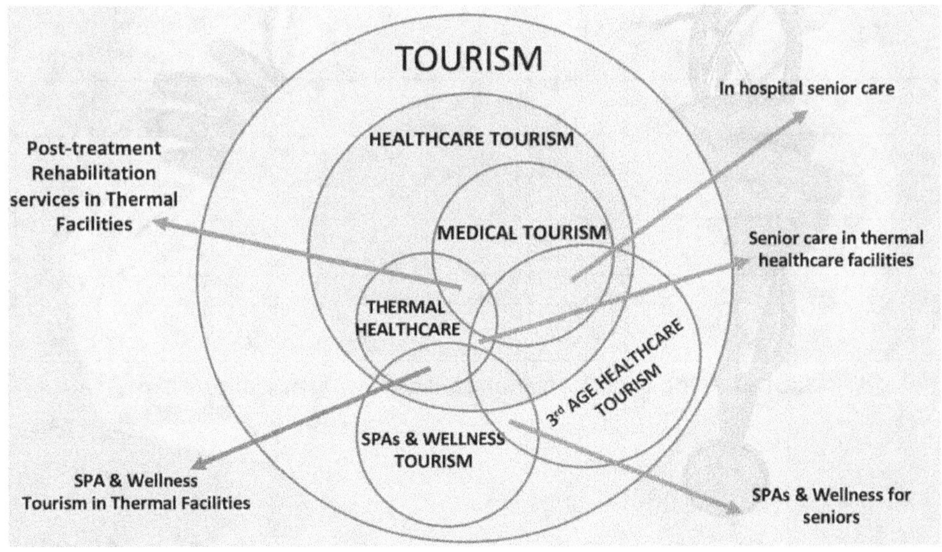

Figure 3 - Relations between tourism-healthcare tourism-medical tourism-thermal healthcare and others

This care "is typically paid for 'out-of-pocket' and is motivated by an interest in cost savings and/or avoiding waiting times for care in the patient's home country".

There is a consensus between different authors to consider medical tourism as a subset of healthcare tourism as shown in Figure 3. Although cross-border mobility occurs for any medical procedure, from simple physical examination to liver transplantation, the treatment or medical procedures listed in Table 7 are the most common reasons for medical tourism.

Main Topics	Sample treatment or procedures
Cosmetic surgeries	Breast augmentation, Face lift Liposuction Hair transplantation
Dentistry	Dental implants Cosmetic and reconstructive procedures
Cardiology/cardiac surgery	By-pass, Valve replacement Angiography Coronary Stenting
Orthopedic surgery	Hip replacement Knee replacement Ankle resurfacing
Oncological	Oncological surgeries Chemotherapies Radiotherapies
Bariatric surgery	gastric by-pass, gastric banding
Transplantation	Liver, Kidney, Lung, Extremity transplantation Cell and tissue transplantation, Stem cell therapies
Fertility/reproductive system	IVF Gender reassignment
Eye surgery	Laser eye surgeries
Others	Diagnostic procedures Check-ups etc.

Table 7 - The most common reasons for medical tourism

In recent years, the ministries of tourism, the ministries of health and entities such as the WHO, the American Medical Association and consultancy firms like Deloitte or PwC have conducted studies indicating awareness of the economic implications of medical tourism to the national economies. The active regions and countries delivering medical tourism services shown in Table 8.

Region	Countries
Asia	Malaysia India Thailand South Korea Singapore
Western Europe	UK Germany
Central Europe	Hungary Croatia Czech Republic
Eastern Europe	Turkey Hungary Poland
Africa	South Africa Tunis
Middle East	UAE Jordan
South and Central America	Costa Rica Mexico Brazil Cuba
North America	USA Canada

Table 8 - Active regions and countries delivering medical tourism services

Patients are increasingly seeking a wide range of medical treatments abroad but complications may occur during medical treatment in a foreign country, which raises medico-legal and insurance matter, as well as anxiety about the follow-up procedures of patients. Physicians need to be ready for counselling, including travel health guidance, to patients seeking cross-border medical treatment.

Insurance, legal and ethical issues in Medical tourism

Medical tourists require special travel insurance policies as regular travel insurance may preclude medical tourism. Many companies now offering travel insurance for medical tourism, which may also assist in the event of any complications of treatment. Travelers should always be advised to check that their travel insurance policy will provide healthcare, emergency assistance. Patients would need to learn medical complaints and legal systems abroad if they wished to take action against a healthcare provider or facility in the event of malpractice. They may find that medical travelers have limited or no protection.

At present, there are no agreed medical complaints or legal frameworks globally to cover medical tourism, except for organ transplantation. The World Health Assembly resolved its objection to organ trafficking and transplant tourism in the form of the Declaration of Istanbul in 2004.34 A number of unethical practices have been described subsequently. In 2006, for example, 4000 prisoners in China were executed to provide 8000 kidneys and 3000 livers, mainly for foreign patients treated with these organs. There is a well-established framework of healthcare ethics promoting the importance of autonomy, including giving informed consent, non-maleficence (benefits should outweigh the risks) and beneficence (promoting patients' welfare and justice). It is likely that medical tourism adds to a two-tiered health system and there may be debates around whether medical tourism benefits the people in the host country.

The use of experimental, unproven or even illegal treatments in medical tourism also raises ethical issues, such as described in relation to stem cell therapies.

The medical tourism sector is expanding rapidly, and people from developed countries as well as investors from all over the world are aware of its future dimensions. Countries such as Thailand, India, Turkey, Malaysia, Costa Rica and Mexico, with some others, have flourishing medical tourism sectors and are attracting medical travellers by the hordes.

Medical tourism is an expectation-driven sector, which is influenced by the complex interaction between medical, economic, social and political forces. Naturally, individuals who are looking for cross-border medical treatment expect similar or better quality of healthcare services (compared to those available in their own countries) without waiting time. The important factors that influence people's decision to become medical travelers are better- personalized care, better hospitality, best hospital design, latest medicines, up-to-date technology, easy transportation, and security. Such additional benefits for patients facilitate their decision to become medical tourists. Table 9 shows intrinsic and extrinsic drivers which are related to medical tourism. Medical tourism is the fact that especially the last quarter-century which cannot be ignored. For a variety of reasons, patients seek treatment options outside their home country. The main factors listed in Table 9 show that health tourism will be an important topic in the future of healthcare delivery. As a matter of fact, when we look at the factors in the table, we can easily say that these reasons are getting stronger day by day both in the favour of push and pull factors.

Intrinsic (Repulsive/Pushing) Factors	Extrinsic (Attractive/Pulling) Factors
Push from the home country	Pull by the destination country
<ul><li>Demographic changes</li><li>High cost of healthcare services</li><li>Poor quality of healthcare services</li><li>Prohibited health services (circumvention)</li><li>Long waiting lists</li><li>Problems on access to care</li><li>Inadequate insurance coverage</li><li>Increased out-of-pocket payments for healthcare</li><li>Health system</li><li>International agreements</li><li>Diaspora effect</li></ul>	<ul><li>Cheaper healthcare service</li><li>No or short waiting list</li><li>Short distance from home country (short flying time)</li><li>High-quality health services and up-to-date technology</li><li>Accredited healthcare provider and reputation of service providers (hospital or doctor)</li><li>Ease of access to care</li><li>Better transportation opportunities</li><li>Organized facilitators</li><li>Cultural closeness and similarities</li><li>Simplified visa formalities</li><li>Communication without language barrier</li><li>Opportunity to visit their homeland</li><li>Destination facts (touristic attractions, historical places)</li><li>Social media and networking</li><li>International agreements</li><li>Diaspora effect</li></ul>

Table 9 - Intrinsic and extrinsic factors in healthcare tourism

The following are the main drivers of medical tourism that will shape the future of healthcare service:

1) Demographic changes: One of the latest reports from the United Nations reveals that the proportion of 65+ year-old people in the populations of developed countries will jump from 17% today to 24% by 2035. The median age of the global population was 29.6 years in 2015, up from 27.5 years a decade earlier. From 2005 to 2015, average life expectancy increased by 3 years and reached 72 years. In the United States, as of 2010, the 'baby boomer' generation has retired, thereby resulting in greater demand for more sophisticated health care. Many US healthcare providers and hospitals are already overwhelmed by the number of patients and the increased demand from baby boomers. In the near future, cross-border health care providers and governments, mostly in developing countries, will develop policies to provide health care to more portion of the growing elderly population.

2) Cost: A direct relationship exists between the health status of the population and the household income. Further, direct and indirect links exist between economic globalization and the determinants of health. As a common feature of medical travel, it is associated with the patients' financial ability to make such a voyage. Economic globalization and cost-cutting policies in the healthcare sector have a direct impact on population health. Owing to the effects of economic changes, especially on cost of living and accompanying limited health insurance policies, individuals are seeking access to lower- priced health care.

Among the developed countries, the US and South Africa do not have national healthcare systems. In the US healthcare system, private health insurance is provided by employers with individual complementarity. In most cases, these insurance plans perform poorly in cost/benefit measures. Although the US is a leading country vis-a-vis treatment modalities, healthcare services and health technology worldwide, Americans pay at least twice for such services, compared to the citizens of many other developed countries. This condition puts a heavy pressure on healthcare financing bodies as well as on insurance companies, healthcare providers, and individuals.

As the economic recession continues to burden people financially, the interest of people in medical tourism is increasing, as a natural corollary. Patients who need medical support have started searching for more affordable medical care at the best price and with acceptable quality. Emerging economies such as India, Turkey, Malaysia, Thailand, and Mexico, have lower living costs; standards of living and salary rates in these countries are far lower than those in developed countries, which is also reflected in prices of healthcare services.

3) Quality: The growth and emergence of any industry, including medical tourism, is directly related to its technological and scientific development. For best medical practice to be conducted most effectively, facilities must be structured in accordance with the latest technological developments in developing countries to support medical tourism. The quality of healthcare services in developing countries has improved through the use of the latest technology. Developing countries have modern facilities along with Western-trained health personnel who provide medical treatment for half of the treatment costs in developed countries. Also, many medical service providers obtain their accreditation certificates from QHA-Trent, JCI, Accreditation Canada or other relevant independent bodies. This encourages patients and insurance companies to seek care from accredited healthcare institutions regardless of their location. The main thematic features of international accreditation standards are focused on patient care services. A basic requirement is to establish a protocol for continuity of healthcare by taking appropriate measures on discharge, dispatch, follow-up, and transfer of patients. Therefore, patients prefer this type of centers to obtain treatment. Patients and insurers know that accredited hospitals in different countries all over the world are operated according to the same exacting standards of developed countries' hospitals. Quality management in such settings could be seen as the professionalization of the medical tourism sector and will attract more patients in the future.

4) Insurance business: The insurance business is globalizing all over the world and in the future health insurance will accept hospitals with certain criteria, without physical border. In the private healthcare sector, insurance companies serve as intermediaries that pay healthcare providers on behalf of healthcare consumers. Private insurance companies and social insurance systems, which have sold health insurance policies to a large number of individuals, have signed contracts with healthcare providers to get "price reduction". The same situation happens in the medical tourism sector. It is natural for insurance companies to use the disparities of prices for medical procedures to their advantage even overseas.

5) Access to care: For patients from countries where governmental healthcare system or private insurance companies control access to services, the major reasons to choose cross-border medical care are to circumvent delays associated with waiting lists or high prices. National healthcare programmes do not typically pay for cosmetic surgery, dental surgery and similar types of services; therefore, patients from the US, Canada and UK who desire these procedures pursue medical tourism for economic reasons. Patients also travel to medical destinations to have procedures that are not widely available in their own countries, such as stem cell therapy, which may be unavailable or restricted in their countries. Circumvention medical tourism occurs when patients travel cross-border to get healthcare services that is "illegal" or "unapproved" in their home countries. Circumvention tourism also has the potential to slow the process of research, as patients go abroad for interventions and opt out of domestic clinical trials. Strict regulations and restrictions on certain procedures such as dilation and curettage (D&C), organ transplantation, surrogacy, IVF with gender selection etc. resulted as circumvention medical tourism as an opportunity of access to care. High-Intensity Focused Ultrasound (HIFU) treatment for prostate cancer, which is approved in Canada and the EU but not the US, is one example. HIFU treatment is performed in the Bahamas by US-based doctors and this is important opportunities for patients seeking such a treatment modality. For patients, the troubles in accessing health care in their own countries supports medical tourism and will continue in the future. Accessible health care in foreign countries also supports medical travel.

6) Waiting time/list: Waiting times in many developed countries, especially those with national healthcare or social insurance systems, are often lengthy and also costly for some surgical procedures. In medical tourism destinations, the waiting time is minimal compared with the patients' own country in elective surgeries such as hip replacement, cholecystectomy and prostatectomy. Developing countries which have medical tourism-targeted policies typically have shorter waiting periods for most of the medical procedures including appointments, surgical operations or checkups. When efficiency and shorter waiting times are combined, countries such as India, Thailand, South Africa, Turkey, Malaysia, Mexico, Singapore and Hungary attract patients from the US and the UK. For example, the waiting time for by-pass surgery or hip replacement surgery in Turkey is only one days. However, in the UK, the waiting time for cataract eye surgery may take as long as two years; this surgery is available without waiting time in many developing countries such as India, Thailand, Turkey and Malaysia. Medical tourism is promoted as a solution to the high price of medical care and as well as treatment delays in USA. In UK and some other publicly funded healthcare driven countries, medical brokerages attract people tired of waiting for hip and knee joint replacement surgeries, cataract surgery and other similar procedures. These will change medical service delivery in future of healthcare.

7) Other drivers of globalisation for future of healthcare

• *Sense and sensibility:* Unfortunately, healthcare services have missed their humanitarian values and become a wild professional business. In most cases, the industry has lost the sensitivity of personal caring and interaction between patients and physicians. Nowadays in busy clinics, a patient is seen as a number rather than as a social individual, and the success rate of clinics or physicians is measured by the income provided to the institution. Many patients feel that surgeons in developed countries are not reachable. Medical tourists who receive treatment abroad share their experiences of personal service and feeling of connection with the healthcare professionals who supervised their treatment. Patients prefer to have physicians whom they can contact with any questions about their clinical situations.

• *Diaspora:* A number of studies have been conducted on a group of medical tourists classified as diaspora travellers. Studies describe this condition in relation to India, China, Korea and Mexico, with recent migrants returning to their countries of origin to access healthcare services. Also, Turkey has a large diasporic population in Europe, and so do countries such as Germany, the Netherlands, France, and Belgium. Some government and medical companies have targeted this group of people and created special programmes for those who have cultural and social similarities or family roots in a medical destination. Diasporic populations targeted by medical tourism programmes are expected to become more popular in the next decade of healthcare. Managing diaspora patients is easy because they travel towards a familiar environment including language and socio-cultural life. Furthermore, most developed nations have large first- and second-generation immigrant populations. This group of people is predisposed to return to their countries of origin for healthcare and will continue in the future. Patients and their relatives prefer their countries of origin because of better communication and the opportunity to visit their relatives at the same time. The medical diaspora has contributed significantly to the medical tourism industry and is becoming increasingly prominent.

• *Medical tourism facilitators:* Medical tourism facilitators are usually organizations operated by medical or tourism sector professionals with technical and medical knowledge. These facilitators usually work with physicians, surgeons, and other medical staff on the basis of the analysis of medical documentation and consultations of patients. They decide which clinic or medical department or hospital is appropriate for future medical travellers. Most of the facilitators have contracts or agreements with healthcare providers in their targeted market countries and they will dominate future of healthcare. They know the capability and quality as well as the rates charged by targeted health service providers.

• *Visa formalities:* The medical travel market is promising. A medical visa is an authentication issued to an individual and set in the individual's travel permit. Patients and relatives are authorized to enter the country for a particular span of time and for the purpose of medical treatment. For example, patients flying to India for medical treatment can get it only for treatment in reputed or accredited hospitals. Up to two attendants who are blood relatives are permitted to go with the patient. Countries such as Germany, USA, UK, Turkey, Malaysia, and India offer quicker and easier travel permit (entry visa) for the patient with certain medical conditions. This is encouraging people for medical tourism.

• *Better transportation opportunities:* Geographical distance, travel time, ease of reaching the destination and location of healthcare providers are key factors in medical tourism. Patients are not willing to experience long-haul indirect flights, tiresome traffic between the airport and the hospital, complicated visa procedures and problematic customs processes. Nowadays, cheaper ticket prices and regular flight schedules provide a faster connection between countries, thereby fostering medical tourism.

• *Better communication opportunities:* Language barriers is a very important disadvantage for medical professionals as well as patients. Hospitals, facilitators and governmental organizations must provide a solution for better communication in patients' mother language.

• *Social media and networking:* Stories and news on similar health services at low prices easily spread globally through social networks. Sharing experiences on social media are powerful marketing tools. Thus, medical tourists are similar to global 'ambassadors' for the destination country and healthcare providers. A large number of websites are advertising healthcare for patients who would like to travel for health reasons. Web search is one of the major tools for gathering information on medical tourism, and it might continue to grow importance by the prospective medical travellers.

• *Destination facts:* The destination's image, reputation, climate, tourist attractions, infrastructure and historical background are factors that influence the perception of patients. These factors have a key role in patients' decision making about countries and hospitals.

• *Health System:* The health status of the population and its distribution throughout the country is directly related to the healthcare system of that country and the health risks faced by the population. The home countries health system plays a significant role in the development of contemporary patient mobility. The concept of medical travel different in the EU than the US. The EU provide healthcare to patients in a controlled manner based on social rights. This is revolutionary and historical epoch-making changes on patient mobility, which began as individuals contesting their right to receive health care in any EU state and resulted in an EU directive on patient rights.

• *International agreements:* Some countries send their expert to other countries for medical procedures or educational purpose. This is an important marketing opportunity for medical tourism destinations. Also, accepting medical students or postgraduate residents from other countries gives opportunities for future collaboration when they returned their homeland. For example, Turkey accepts students from Balkan countries and from many African countries for almost 30 years, depending on agreements. When students return back to the homeland, their medical teachers are acting as a consultant for them in any need of expert opinion. In further, if patient needs to be referred to a cross-border country their medical school takes first places. Also, Turkey signed international agreements with many countries to accept patients for certain medical procedures such as oncological or cardiovascular surgeries.

Conclusion

International rules related to medical tourism need to be developed and implemented. However, the potential effects of medical tourism on the healthcare sector and other related sectors should not be ignored. This condition demonstrates the need to assess the full health impact of international agreements to be formulated. Educated consumers, a growing middle class, well-trained physicians, high-technology healthcare institutions and struggling public healthcare systems are some of the forces behind the demand for medical tourism. New healthcare and globalized economic policies are unable to meet the needs and expectations of patients, thereby forcing the globalization of healthcare. Evidently, medical tourism is an emerging multi-dimensional sector with effects on the healthcare system of developed and developing countries. Consequently, medical tourism, which refers to the cross-border mobilization of healthcare services, is operating with the expectation that healthcare services will be validated through accreditation of quality and safety measurement systems with proven standards.

The growth of the sector depends on local government bodies, policies, the power of private healthcare sector, airlines, travel agents, medical tourism facilitators and hotels working together as well as government-supported marketing to promote medical tourism. This sector has significant impacts on doctors, patients, employers, insurance companies, the transportation sector, healthcare providers and policymakers. In their conference paper Kumar et al noticed eleven independent factors for Malaysia such as 'Functions of Responsible State Organizations', 'Functions of Health Centers', 'Cooperation of Responsible Organizations', 'Diversity and Variance of Medical Services', 'Quality of Medical Services', 'Pricing of Medical Services', 'Advertising the Medical Services', 'Geography', 'Security', 'As an Islamic State' and 'Attractions of Medical Tourism Issues'.

Some researchers noted that price transparency and demonstrated savings, accreditation by the JCI or its equivalent, board-certified physicians in the relevant specialties, and an ability and willingness to collaborate with domestic physicians to coordinate before and after voyage care are essential for medical tourism. Regarding some researcher, there are five key drivers of medical tourism, including technological improvements, the cost of the care, the emergence of the new consumer needs, the opportunity to engage in attractive tourism which is certainly a better change for patient and demographic drivers such as aging population. Gill and Singh found five important factors that affect the choice of destination. These are "medical facilities and services", "local primary doctor's recommendation", and "governmental policies and laws" were among the most important choices. The two choices that were relatively important were "hotels and food/beverage quality" and "general tourism supply" of destination.

Patients are traveling beyond borders in search of affordable and timely healthcare services. Many medical tourism facilitating companies are now involved in organizing and arranging crossborder health services. Despite the rapid expansion of the medical tourism industry, few standards exist to ensure that these businesses organize highquality, competent international healthcare.

Final Words:

This chapter has explored as much information as possible to present an overall view of the key factors that influence medical tourism. Studies on healthcare tourism have attracted close scrutiny because most of the available articles are qualitative. Most of the information on medical tourism is Web-based or published in magazines. Also, many academic journals have published studies or reports of quantitative findings on medical tourism. Today, reforms related to the healthcare system are ongoing in many countries. Thus, the evaluations presented in this study are valuable for those who work at all stages of the reform process.

In a global manner, the quantity of medical travel and its service-related economic dimensions is still limited, when compared with total health expenditures. Currently, issues of cross-border social security, the cross-border mobility of patients and services are of special relevance for touristic regions, regions attracting retired persons, and both sides' border zones neighborhoods. However, the question of how and which economic and political dynamics in the future of healthcare will shape cross-border patients' mobility remains open.

References
1. Bennie R (2014). Medical Tourism: A Look at How Medical Outsourcing Can Reshape Health Care, Texas International Law Journal Vol. 49:583-600
2. Carrera, P., & Bridges, J. (2006a). Globalization and healthcare: understanding health and medical tourism. Expert Review of Pharmacoeconomics and Outcomes Research, 6 (Suppl 4), 447-454,
3. Connell, J. (2006). Medical tourism: Sea, sun, sand and surgery. Tourism Management, 27(6), 1093- 1100, doi:10.1016/j.tourman.2005.11.005.
4. Connell J, (2013): Contemporary medical tourism: Conceptualisation, culture and commodification, Tourism Management, Volume 34, Pages 1-13
5. Crooks VA, Kingsbury P, Snyder J, Johnston R. What is known about the patient's experience of medical tourism? A scoping study. BMC Health Serv Res 2010;10:266.
6. Delmonico FL. The implications of Istanbul Declaration on organ trafficking and transplant tourism. Curr Opin Organ Transplant 2009; 14:116–19.
7. Euromonitor International (2017); Old Is the New Young: How Global Consumers Are Challenging Ageing, Retrieved from http://go.euromonitor.com/rs/805-KOK-   719/images/sbOldNewYoungGlobalConsumersChallengingAgeing.pdf (accessed: 23 July 2019)
8. Euromonitor International (2017); Old Is the New Young: How Global Consumers Are Challenging Ageing, Retrieved on 23 July 2019 http://go.euromonitor.com/rs/805-KOK-719/images/sbOldNewYoungGlobal-ConsumersChallengingAgeing.pdf
9. Gill H, Singh N, (2011), Exploring the Factors that Affect the Choice of Destination for Medical Tourism, Journal of Service Science and Management, 2011, 4, 315-324
10. HOPE - European Hospital and Healthcare Federation, Medical Tourism report; 2015, Retrieved on 22 August 2017 http://www.hope.be/wp-content/uploads/2011/15/98_2015_HOPE-PUBLICATION_Medical-Tourism.pdf
11. Horowitz MD., Rosensweig JA., Jones CA., (2007) Medical Tourism: Globalization of the Healthcare Marketplace, MedGenMed. 2007; 9(4): 33. Retrieved on 22 July 2018 https://www.ncbi.nlm.nih.gov/pmc/articles/PMC2234298/
12. Jagyasi, D.P. (2008). Defining Medical Tourism. Retrieved on 2 September 2018,   http://www.medicaltourismmag.com/defining-medical-tourism-another-approach/
13. Khan M, "Medical Tourism: Outsourcing of Healthcare" (2010). International CHRIE Conference-Refereed Track. 23. Retrieved on 22 August 2017, http://scholarworks.umass.edu/refereed/CHRIE_2010/Friday/23
14. Kumar J, Hussian K, Shahi M (2012). The Proceedings of 11th Asia Pacific Forum for Graduate Students Research in Tourism and International Convention and Expo Summit 2012, 22-24 May 2012 Hong Kong SAR, China; Retrieved on 9 September 2018,   https://www.researchgate.net/publication/273317674_An_Evaluation_of_the_Factors_for_Medical_Tourism_Destination_Selection
15. Lunt N, Smith R, Exworthy M, et al. Medical tourism: treatments, markets and health system implications: a scoping review. OECD, Directorate for Employment, labour and Social Affairs, 2011. Available at www.oecd.org/ els/health-systems/48723982.pdf Retrieved on 4 November 2018.
16. Lunt N, Smith RD, Mannion R, Green ST, Exworthy M, Hanefeld J, et al (2014). Implications for the NHS of inward and outward medical tourism: a policy and economic analysis using literature review and mixed-methods approaches. Health Serv Deliv Res; 2 (2); 16-17.

17. Lunt N, Horsfall DG, Hanefeld J, (2016); Medical tourism: A snapshot of evidence on treatment abroad. Maturitas. pp. 37-44. ISSN 0378-5122

18. Mainil T, Van Loon F, Botterill D, Dinnie K, Platenkamp V, Meulemans H, (2012), Framing and Measuring International Patient Management, in Leonard H. Friedman, Grant T. Savage, Jim Goes (ed.) Annual Review of Health Care Management: Strategy and Policy Perspectives on Reforming Health Systems (Advances in Health Care Management, Volume 13) Emerald Group Publishing Limited, pp.145 – 159

19. Mestrovic T. (2014), Retrieved on 22 August 2018, http://www.news-medical.net/health/Medical-Tourism-Accreditation.aspx

20. Munro JW (2012). "What is medical tourism? Retrieved on 22 August 2018 http://www.globalwellnesssummit.com/wp-content/uploads/Industry-Research/Global/2012-mtqa-what-is-medical-tourism.pdf

21. Rollyson S; Drivers, Business Drivers of Medical Tourism, Retrieved on 23 August 2018, http://globalizationhealthcare.net/analysis/drivers/

22. SFU Medical Tourism Research Group (2015); Did you know...? A fact sheet about medical tourism; Circumvention Medical Tourism; Simon Fraser University Medical Tourism Research Group. Retrieved on 29 August 2018 http://www.sfu.ca/medicaltourism/One%20page%20summaries%20June%202015/Circumvention%20Medical%20Tourism.pdf

23. Tontus HO, Nebioglu S (2018); Drivers of Healthcare Globalisation and Their Effects on Medical Tourism, e-Review of Tourism Research (eRTR), Vol. 15, No. 2-3, 2018

24. Turner LG (2010). "Medical tourism" and the global marketplace in health services: U.S. patients, international hospitals, and the search for affordable health care; International Journal of Health Services, Volume 40, Number 3, Pages 443–467

25. Turner LG (2011). Quality in Health Care and Globalization of Health Services: Accreditation and Regulatory Oversight of Medical Tourism Companies Int J Qual Health Care. 23(1):17

26. Woodward D, Drager N, Beaglehole R, Lipson D (2001). Globalization and health: a framework for analysis and action, Bulletin of the World Health Organization, 79 (9), 875-881

FUTURE
of HEALTHCARE

Chai CHUAH & Dr H. Omer TONTUS